Digestive System - Recent Advances

Edited by Xingshun Qi and Sam Koruth

Published in London, United Kingdom

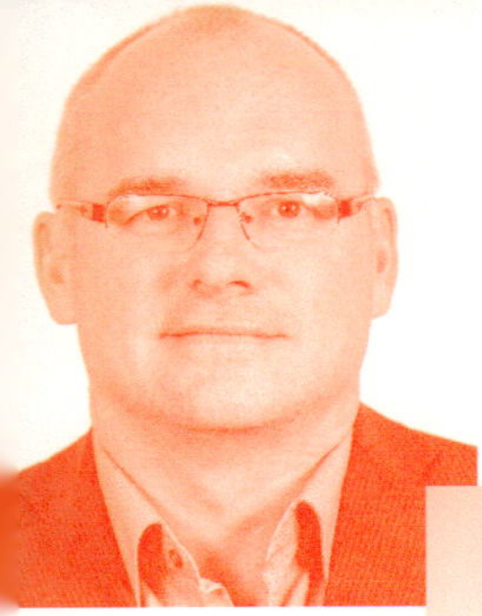
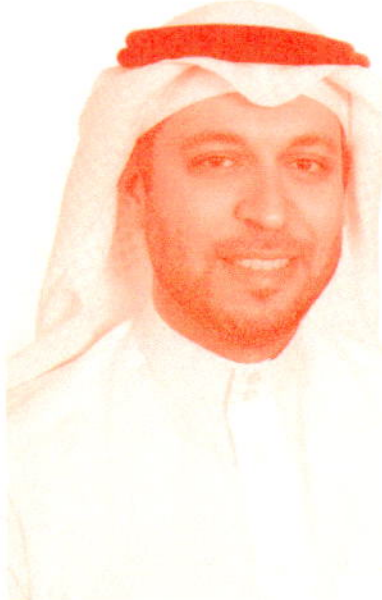
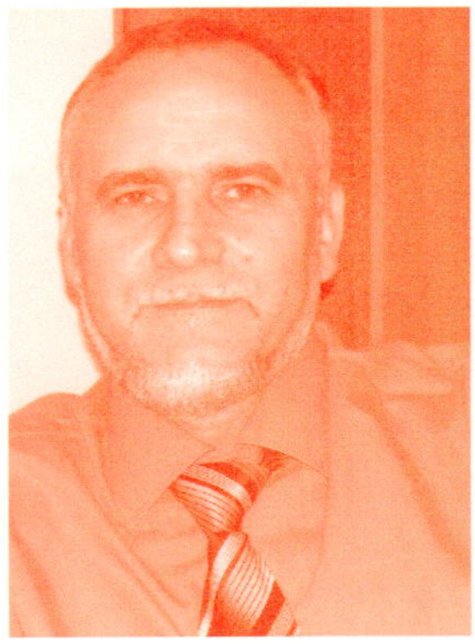
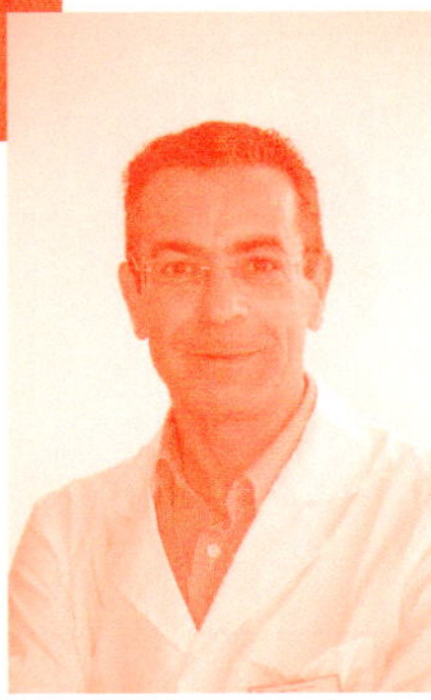
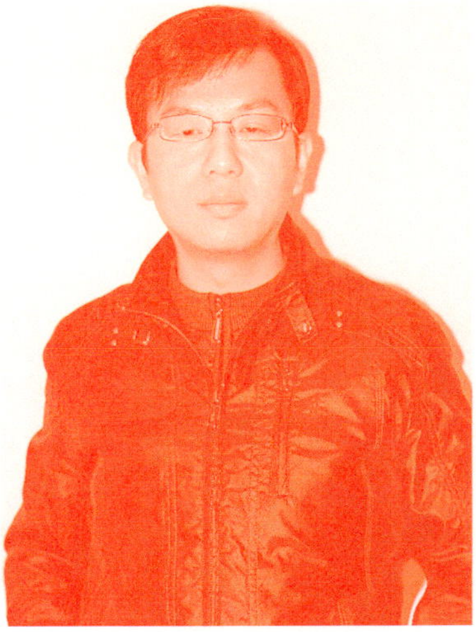
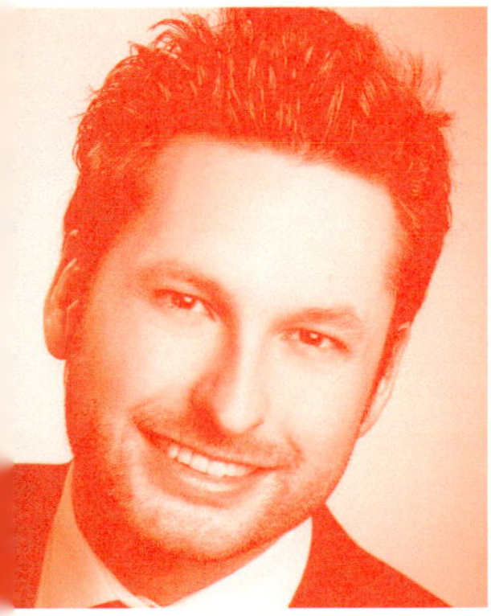
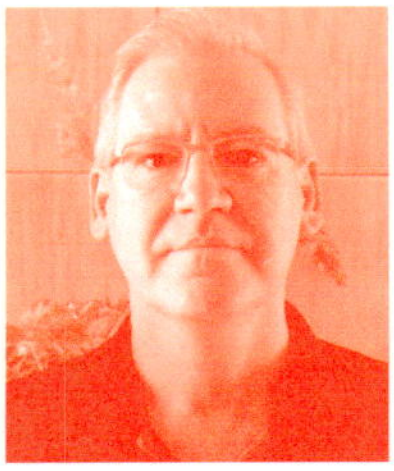

IntechOpen

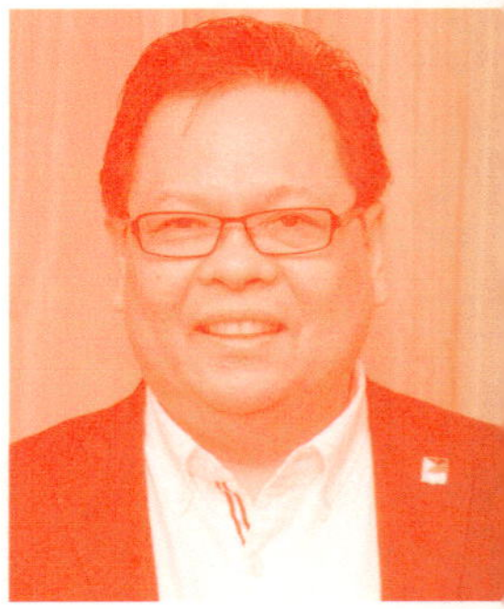
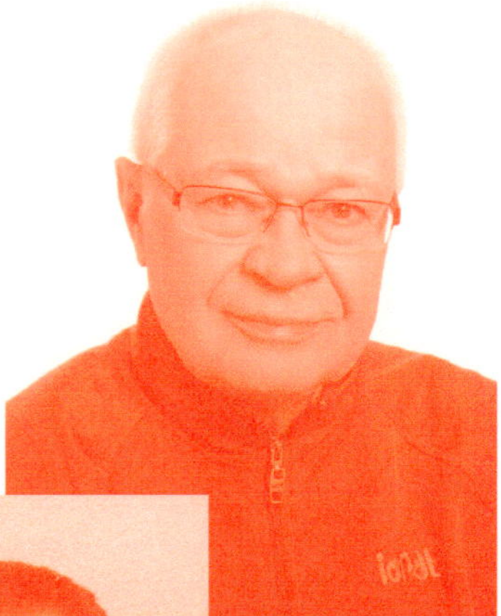
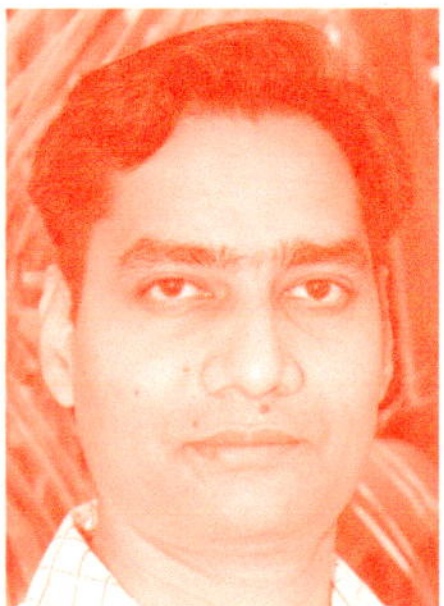
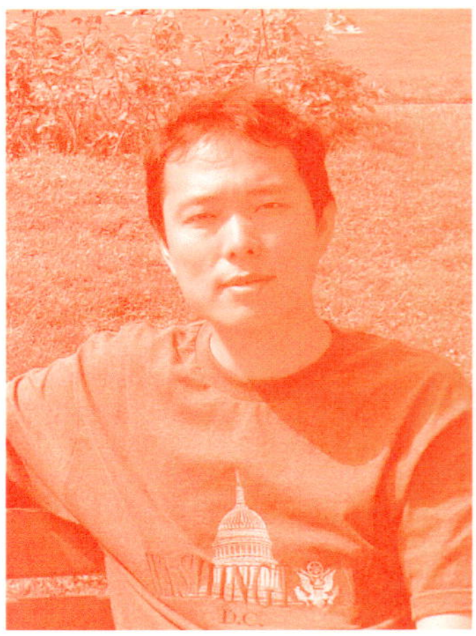
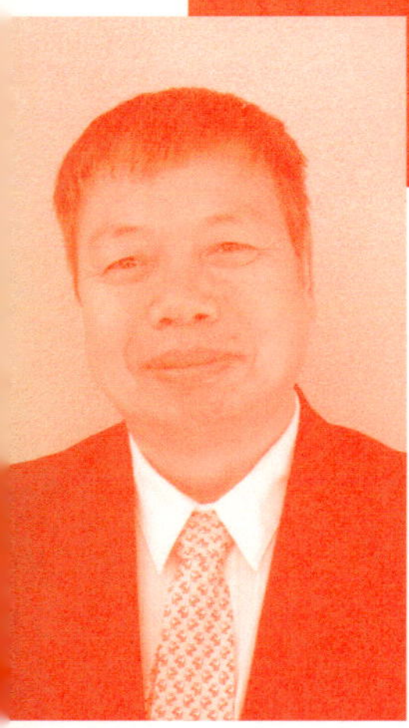
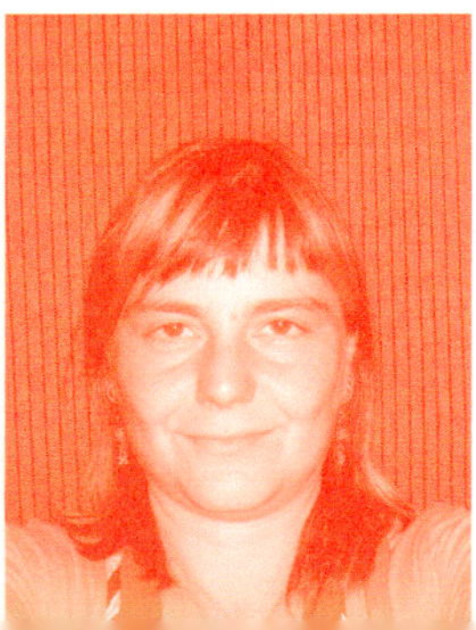

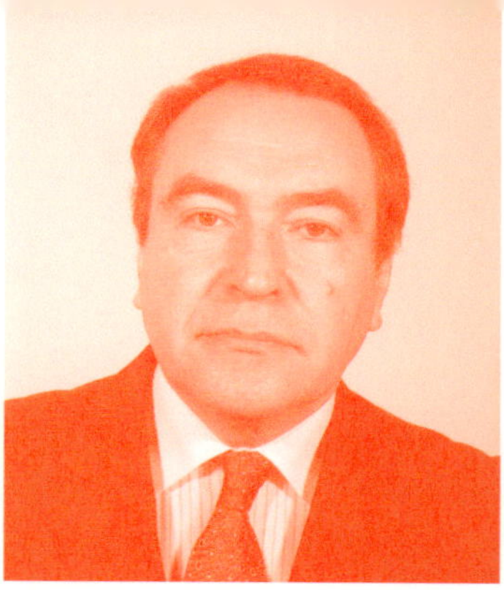
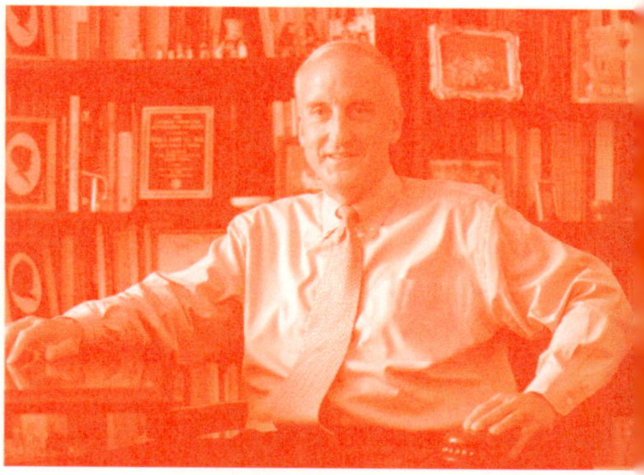
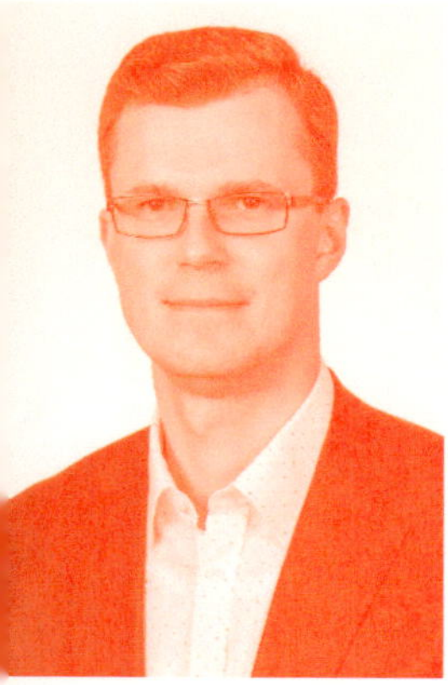
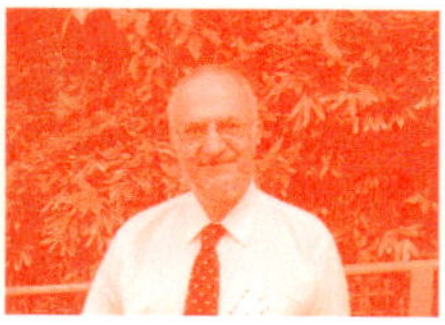
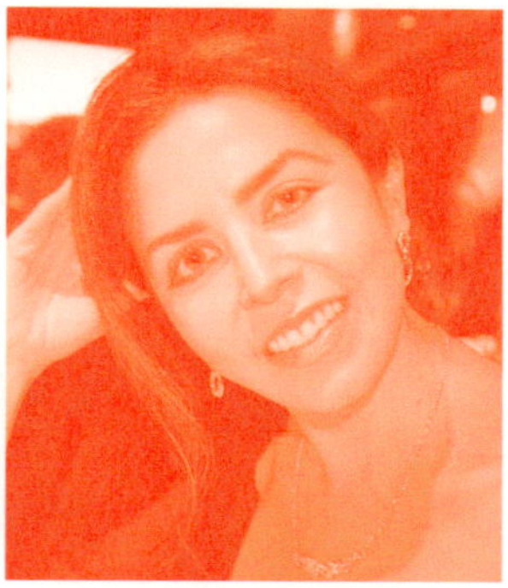

Supporting open minds since 2005

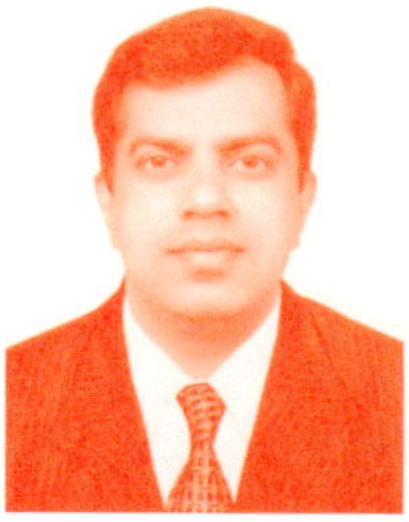
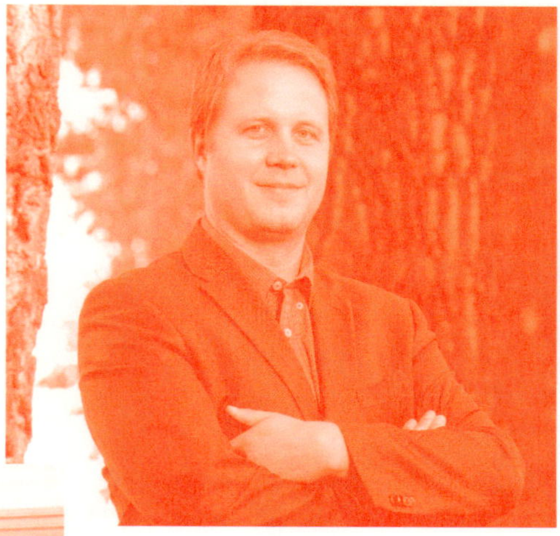
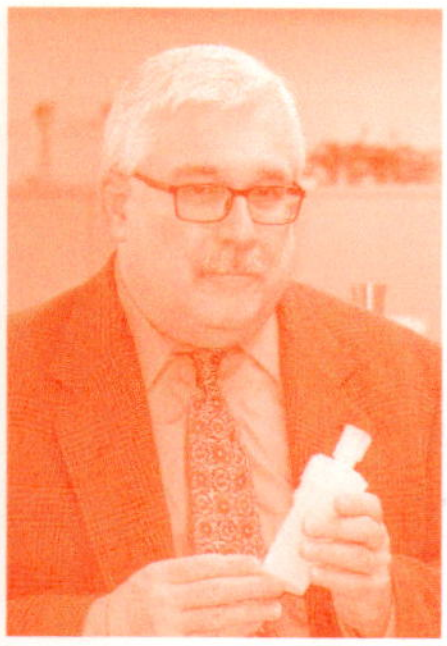
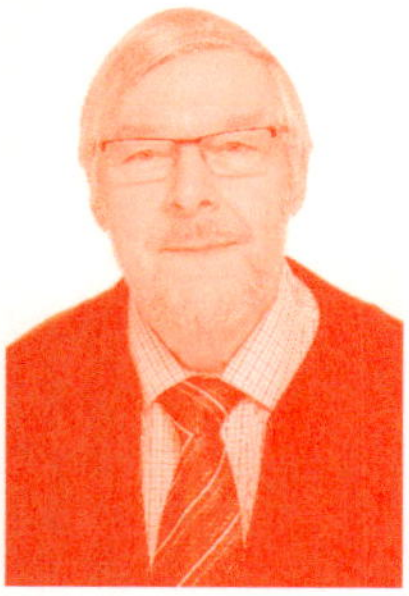
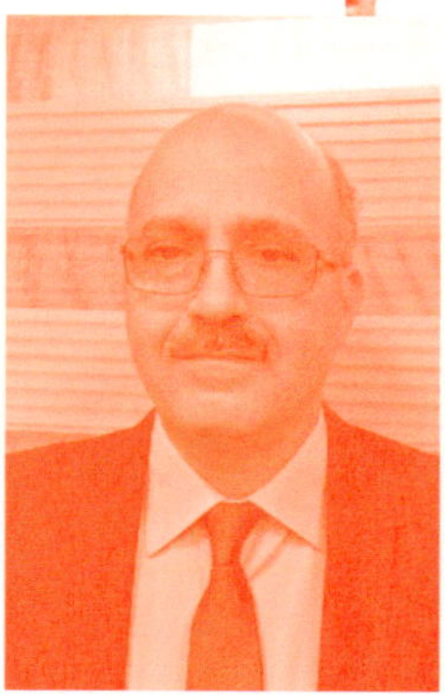
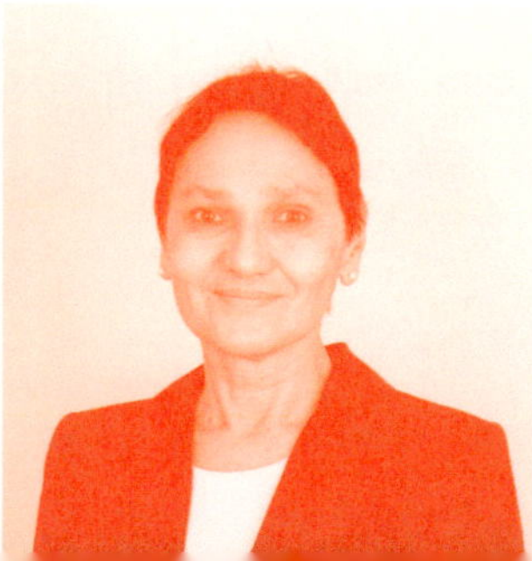
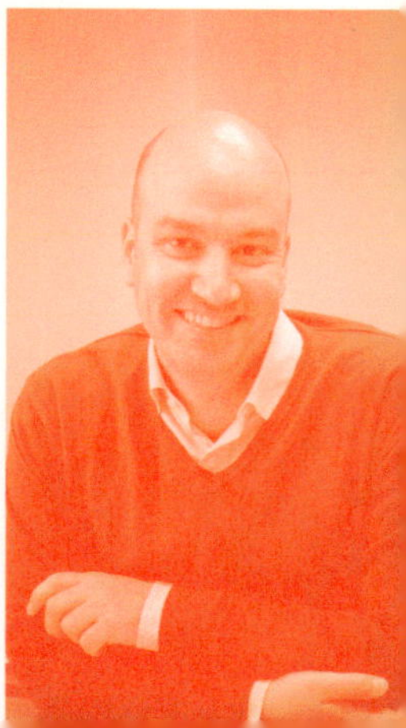

Digestive System - Recent Advances
http://dx.doi.org/10.5772/intechopen.77789
Edited by Xingshun Qi and Sam Koruth

Contributors
Ahmed Elgeidie, Toshifumi Wakai, Pankaj Prasoon, Tomohiro Katada, Jun Sakata, Yuki Hirose, Wala Ben Kridis, Nabil Toumi, Jamel Daoud, Afef Khanfir, Mounir Frikha, Camelia Cojocariu, Ana Maria Singeap, Stefan Chiriac, Catalin Sfarti, Irina Girleanu, Oana Petrea, Anca Trifan, Carol Stanciu, Monjur Ahmed, Ravi Kant Avvari, Xingshun Qi, Sam Koruth

First published in London, United Kingdom, 2020 by IntechOpen
IntechOpen is the global imprint of INTECHOPEN LIMITED, registered in England and Wales, registration number: 11086078, 7th floor, 10 Lower Thames Street, London, EC3R 6AF, United Kingdom
Printed in Croatia

British Library Cataloguing-in-Publication Data
A catalogue record for this book is available from the British Library

Additional hard and PDF copies can be obtained from orders@intechopen.com

Digestive System - Recent Advances
Edited by Xingshun Qi and Sam Koruth
p. cm.
Print ISBN 978-1-78985-139-7
Online ISBN 978-1-78985-140-3
eBook (PDF) ISBN 978-1-83968-390-9

For EU product safety concerns:
IN TECH d.o.o., Prolaz Marije Krucifikse Kozulić 3, 51000 Rijeka, Croatia, info@intechopen.com or visit our website at intechopen.com.

Meet the editors

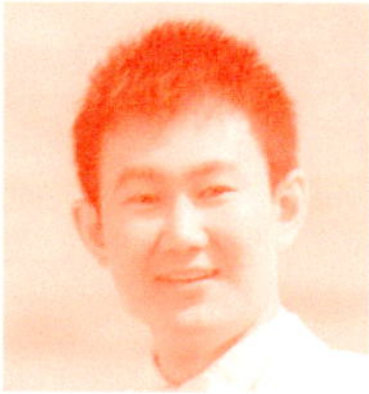

Dr. Xingshun Qi was born in July 1984 in Shenyang, obtained his doctoral degree at the Fourth Military Medical University in Xi'an, and completed his post-doctoral fellowship at the General Hospital of Shenyang Military Area in Shenyang, China. He is currently working at the Department of Gastroenterology of the General Hospital of Shenyang Military Area as a Vice Chief Physician. His major work was published in the *Nature Reviews Gastroenterology and Hepatology, BMC Medicine, Journal of Hepatology, Clinical Gastroenterology and Hepatology, Alimentary Pharmacology & Therapeutics, Thrombosis and Haemostasis, American Journal of Medicine,* etc. He has edited one English-language book and written several chapters for 7 English and Chinese books. He has served as a peer-reviewer in more than 110 journals. According to the Scopus, his H-index is 32, and total number of citation is 3185.

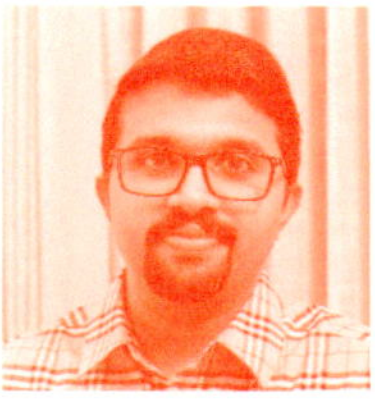

Dr. Sam Koruth's educational qualifications include MBBS, MS (General Surgery), FMAS, and DMAS (Fellowship and Diploma in Minimal Access Surgery). He has worked in the field of general surgery for over 6 years, and is currently practicing in Lourdes Hospital Kochi, Kerala, India where he has been trained under the reputed surgeon Dr. Santhosh John Abraham (Former President of Associations of Surgeons of India). In the last 6 years, Dr. Koruth has presented various papers at national and state levels and has published many articles in the international forum. He also got the privilege of co-editing two chapters in the book "Contemporary Book of Surgery". Dr. Koruth won the *Best Thesis of the Year Award*, the *Best Poster of the Year Award*, *2nd Best Research Paper* and *Best Faculty Video Presentation* in 2017 in the state forum. Additionally, he has won many awards at the national level. His best work has been on "Collagen 3 involvement in all types of Hernias" proving that it's not just a primary disorder but a congenital defect, which has been accepted in an international journal.

Contents

Preface

As a physician working in the Department of Gastroenterology, I am very pleased to cooperate with IntechOpen to launch a book about the digestive system in January 2019. Through persistent efforts, a total of 9 chapters, which are authored by worldwide experts in the field of liver diseases, are included in this book entitled as "***Digestive System - Recent Advances***". The book is divided into 3 major sections: gastrointestinal duct, liver, and biliary system. In more detail, the book covers peptic ulcers, mid-gastrointestinal bleeding, gastrointestinal manifestations of IgA vasculitis, biomechanics of intestinal contractions, gallbladder carcinoma, ERCP for cholecysto-choledocholithiasis, and cystic artery variations and associated vascular complications in laparoscopic cholecystectomy and the evaluation of serum sodium change after terlipressin in cirrhosis. The knowledge presented in the book should be valuable for family physicians, internists, gastroenterologists, and hepatologists who are interested in digestive diseases to guide the clinical practice and management. This book should be also useful for patients and their relatives to better understand the digestive system.

I am deeply indebted to the assistance from IntechOpen staff, including Andrea Koric (Commissioning Editor) and Lada Bozic (Author Service Manager). Also, I greatly appreciate the support from all chapter authors. Finally, I wish to dedicate this book to my wife Jun Liu.

Dr. Xingshun Qi
Department of Gastroenterology,
General Hospital of Northern Theater Command,
China

I am extremely pleased to work with IntechOpen to launch this book on the digestive system, with the section on the biliary system under my supervision. The chapters cover the variations, complications, and latest modifications in various topics of the biliary system. Some of the topics such as gallbladder carcinoma, ERCP for cholecysto-choledocholithiasis, and cystic artery variations and associated vascular complications in laparoscopic cholecystectomy, have been described keeping in mind the current practice and the recent advances in the field. The knowledge presented in this book should be valuable for young surgeons as a guide for the clinical practice and management.

As an editor I have tried to ensure that the descriptions and techniques illustrated are representative of contemporary practice while keeping the information current and simple.

I would like to thank God Almighty for giving me the vision and opportunity to be part of this book. I deeply appreciate the IntechOpen staff, including Andrea Koric (Commissioning Editor) and Lada Bozic (Author Service Manager) for their continuous support. I extend my thanks to all the authors for their time and effort. My sincere gratitude to Dr. Santhosh John Abraham (Professor and HOD Gen Surgery, Past President – Associations of Surgeons of India, Dr. Vimal Iype (Head of Vascular Surgery), my colleagues Dr. Arunesh Dubey, Dr.Nidhin, and Dr. Sooraj Sankar for their timeless help and support. Finally I would like to thank my parents, and my wife for the enormous support throughout the years.

Dr. Sam Koruth
Lourdes Hopital,
Kerala, India

Section 1

Gastrointestinal Duct

Chapter 1

Peptic Ulcer Disease

Monjur Ahmed

Abstract

Peptic ulcer disease (PUD) is one of the commonest diseases seen throughout the world. There are various risk factors for the development of peptic ulcer disease, but the most important ones are *Helicobacter pylori* infection and nonsteroidal anti-inflammatory drugs (NSAIDs). Patients generally present with dyspepsia or peptic ulcer bleeding. Acid suppressant therapy, *H. pylori* eradication, and avoidance of nonsteroidal anti-inflammatory drugs are the cornerstones of treatment of peptic ulcer disease. Peptic ulcer bleeding could be life-threatening. It is managed by appropriate supportive care, intravenous proton pump inhibitor therapy, and endoscopic hemostasis. Transarterial embolization (TAE) and surgery are rarely required if endoscopic therapy fails.

Keywords: peptic ulcer disease, dyspepsia, *H. pylori* infection, peptic ulcer bleeding, endoscopic treatment of peptic ulcer bleeding

1. Introduction

Peptic ulcer disease (PUD) is defined as the mucosal break of the upper gastrointestinal tract due to acid peptic digestion resulting in ulcer formation which extends beyond the muscularis mucosae into the submucosa. Most commonly it occurs in the stomach and first part of the duodenum but can also occur in the distal esophagus, distal duodenum, and jejunum and in the Meckel's diverticulum with heterotrophic gastric mucosa [1]. The size of the ulcer varies from 5 mm to several centimeters. On the other hand, erosions are superficial, less than 5 mm in size, and limited to the mucosa. PUD is still one of the commonest disorders we encounter in our clinical practice. The term "peptic" comes from the hormone pepsin which plays an important role in causing mucosal break. Peptic ulcer (PU) bleeding is the most common cause of upper gastrointestinal bleeding in the western world [2] and results in significant morbidity, mortality, and healthcare costs [3]. PUD is a benign condition, is easily treatable by medical therapy, and rarely requires surgery.

2. Epidemiology

PUD affects about 4.5 million persons per year in the United States (US) and causes huge healthcare cost of about $3.3. billion/year [4]. The prevalence of PUD varies with the prevalence of *Helicobacter pylori* (*H. pylori*) infection. In the United States, the seroprevalence of *H. pylori* infection varies with age: 16.7% in young age (20–29 years) group and 56.9% in older age (>70 years) group. It is also different among different ethnicities: non-Hispanic whites 26.2%, non-Hispanic blacks 52.7%, and Mexican Americans 61.6% [5]. In developing countries, the prevalence of infection can be as high as 90% [6]. Systematic review of the literature from developed countries estimated that the global incidence and prevalence of physician-diagnosed PUD were 0.10–0.19% and 0.12–1.50%, respectively. But the incidence and prevalence of PUD have decreased with the universal use of acid suppressant therapy and decrease in prevalence of *Helicobacter pylori* infection due to improved socioeconomic status and eradication of *H. pylori* infection after detection [7].

3. Etiopathogenesis

H. pylori infection and nonsteroidal anti-inflammatory drugs (NSAIDs) account for majority of the cases of PUD. More than 90% of duodenal ulcers and >70% of gastric ulcers are *H. pylori* positive [8]. A prospective study from Turkey found that *H. pylori* infection alone was responsible for PUD in 75% of cases, both *H. pylori* infection and NSAIDs in 50% of cases and NSAIDs alone in 10% of cases [9]. A Japanese study showed that the long-term use of low-dose aspirin could cause PUD in 6.2% of cases. The risk is increased in diabetic patients and in patients taking anticoagulants [9]. Both NSAIDs and aspirin inhibit the cyclooxygenase pathway and decrease the production of prostaglandin which is responsible for cytoprotection of gastric mucosa by stimulating mucus and bicarbonate secretion and increasing mucosal blood flow [10]. The chance of developing NSAID-induced PUD increases in the presence of certain risk factors which include age more than 65, heart disease, past history of PUD, and co-administration of corticosteroid, antiplatelets, and anticoagulants [11]. All NSAIDs can cause gastrointestinal injuries which include inflammation, erosions, ulcerations, and bleeding. The relative risk varies: the highest risk is associated with piroxicam and ketorolac; high risk with indomethacin and naproxen; intermediate risk with meloxicam, diclofenac, and ketoprofen; and low risk with ibuprofen and celecoxib [12]. About 11% of the US population take NSAIDs on a regular basis. 15–30% of them have PUD on endoscopy although clinical upper gastrointestinal events can occur in 1.5–4.5% of patients taking NSAIDs [13].

H. pylori virulence factors are important in the pathogenesis of PUD. Cytotoxin-associated gene A (Cag A), vacuolating cytotoxin A (Vac A), and induced by contact with epithelium antigen (ice A) are associated with PUD. After entering the stomach, *H. pylori* utilizes its urease enzyme to neutralize the gastric acidity. *H. pylori* then moves toward the gastric epithelium where it binds to the gastric epithelial cell receptors by its adhesion molecule [14]. Cag A is a strong immunogenic protein and measures the virulence of *H. pylori* infection. Cag A gene increases production of IL-8 and activates nuclear factor-kB [15], and ice A increases mucosal IL-8 expression. Gastric epithelial layer then activates its innate immunity and neutrophils leading to gastritis and peptic ulcer formation. Vac A toxin is a pore-forming toxin, and it not only stimulates vacuole formation in gastric epithelial cells, parietal cells, T cells, and other immune cells but also helps *H. pylori* in colonizing the stomach [16].

How H. pylori can cause duodenal ulcer while residing in the gastric mucus layer? In *H. pylori* gastritis, the cytokine tumor necrosis factor inhibits somatostatin cells (D cells) in the antral mucosa. As a result, gastrin secretion becomes uninhibited, leading to hypergastrinemia, hyperacidity, and duodenal ulcer formation [17]. Another study suggests that gastric metaplasia and *H. pylori* colonization in the duodenal bulb could play a critically important role in the pathogenesis of duodenal ulcer [18]. The gastric metaplasia becomes inflamed by *H. pylori* infection which disrupts mucosal regeneration leading to duodenal ulcer formation [19].

There are certain *unusual causes of PUD* which we come across now and then in our clinical practice.

Gastrinoma or Zollinger-Ellison syndrome may present as multiple gastric and duodenal ulcers and accounts for 0.1% or more cases of PUD [20]. Other hormone (histamine)-mediated PUD include systemic mastocytosis, polycythemia vera, and basophilia in myeloproliferative diseases [21].

Besides NSAIDs and low-dose aspirin, few other medications can cause PUD. These include clopidogrel (in combination with NSAIDs), corticosteroids (in combination with NSAIDs), bisphosphonates, potassium chloride, spironolactone, sirolimus, mycophenolate mofetil, hepatic artery infusion of 5-fluorouracil, and selective serotonin reuptake inhibitors [22].

PUD can be due to another helicobacter infection called *Helicobacter heilmannii* [23]. Gastrointestinal ulcerations due to cytomegalovirus, herpes simplex virus, gastric and duodenal tuberculosis, and syphilis can mimic PUD.

Certain infiltrative diseases like Crohn's disease and sarcoidosis can present like PUD [24].

Family history is an independent risk factor for the development of PUD [25]. Blood group O individuals have higher susceptibility of getting *H. pylori* infection [26] and are 35–40% more prone to develop duodenal ulcer than people with other blood groups [27]. Salivary secretory status of A, B, and H antigens was also found to be significant. Nonsecretor phenotypes of ABH antigens are more susceptible to develop *H. pylori* infection and duodenal ulcer [28]. Genetic influence on the formation of PUD is modest, and it is independent of the genetic susceptibility of acquiring *H. pylori* infection [29]. Other risk factors for the development of PUD include smoking and psychological stress [30].

When we think about the pathogenesis of PUD, we must consider two factors:

1. Mucosal protective factors: gastric mucus layer, prostaglandin, bicarbonate, and mucosal blood flow.

2. Mucosal damaging factors: gastric acidity, pepsin, *H. pylori* infection, and NSAIDs.

PU occurs when there is an imbalance between these factors.

3.1 Clinical features

Patients with PUD may be symptomatic or asymptomatic. Symptomatic patients generally present with dyspepsia, i.e., upper abdominal pain or discomfort. Most of the time, the pain is felt in the epigastric region, but sometimes it can be in the right upper quadrant or left upper quadrant of the abdomen. The pain is burning, gnawing, or dull aching in nature and generally non-radiating but rarely can radiate to the back in the case of posterior penetrating ulcer. Patients with gastric ulcer may feel pain shortly after taking food, but in the case of duodenal ulcer, pain is generally felt 2–3 h after taking meal, or sometimes patients wake up at night with epigastric pain. Duodenal ulcer pain is generally relieved after taking antacids or food which has minimal effect on relieving gastric ulcer pain [31]. Sometimes patients may feel gas and bloating sensation in the abdomen and sometimes may experience nausea and vomiting. About 30% of elderly patients with PUD may remain asymptomatic [32]. This is also common in patients taking NSAIDs. Silent PU generally presents with gastrointestinal bleeding [33].

Physical examination can be entirely normal except epigastric tenderness.

3.2 Diagnosis and evaluation

A thorough history and physical examination is necessary to evaluate the patient. In each case, we should look for alarm features which include [34]:

1. Evidence of overt or occult gastrointestinal bleeding: hematemesis, melena, anemia, heme-positive stool

2. Iron deficiency anemia

3. Dysphagia

4. Left supraclavicular lymphadenopathy (Virchow's nodes)

5. Palpable abdominal mass

6. Symptom of impending perforation: severe persistent epigastric pain

7. Symptom of obstruction: persistent vomiting

8. Malignancy: anorexia, unintended weight loss

9. Age: >55 years

Diagnostic tests should include complete blood count, esophagogastroduodenoscopy (EGD), or upper gastrointestinal (UGI) series and tests for detection *H. pylori* infection. EGD is preferred over UGI series as it has much higher diagnostic yield and mucosal biopsy can be taken. Endoscopic views of clean-based duodenal ulcer and gastric ulcer are shown in **Figures 1** and **2**. During endoscopy, the location, size, depth, and any sign or stigmata of bleeding can be evaluated, and gastric biopsy from antrum, body, and incisura can be taken to detect *H. pylori* infection [35]. Although endoscopic evaluation is the gold standard of diagnosis of PUD, it is not cost-effective to perform EGD in all suspected cases of PUD. The

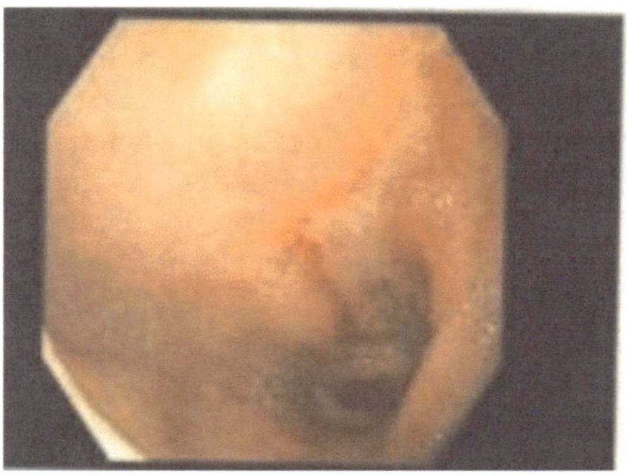

Figure 1.
Duodenal ulcer.

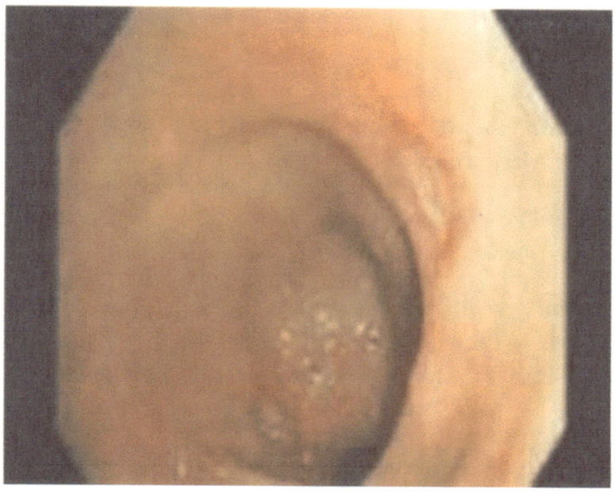

Figure 2.
Gastric ulcers.

alternative non-endoscopic strategies can be considered in the absence of alarm features:

1. *H. pylori* test and treat: In a population where the prevalence of *H. pylori* infection exceeds 20%, patients should get tested for *H. pylori* infection and, if positive, should be treated by anti-*H. pylori* therapy [36, 37]. If *H. pylori* test is negative or patients still remain symptomatic after anti-*H. pylori* therapy, they should be given a 4–6 week course of proton pump inhibitor (PPI) therapy. If PPI therapy fails, patients should be reassured, diagnosis should be reassessed, and EGD should be considered. If patients respond to anti-*H. pylori* treatment or PPI therapy, they can be managed without further investigation [38].

Stool for *H. pylori antigen* and urea breath tests are most accurate not only for identification of active *H. pylori* infection but also for confirmation of eradication of infection. Serology for *H. pylori* antibody is less reliable and cannot be used for confirmation of cure.

2. Empiric acid suppression therapy: In a population where the prevalence of *H. pylori* infection is 10% or less, empiric PPI therapy is most cost-effective. In case of PPI failure, test-and-treat strategy should be applied as mentioned above [39].

Physicians should make decision between test-and-treat strategy and empiric PPI therapy for 4–6 weeks in the absence of alarm features. EGD should be considered in the presence of alarm features. The American College of Gastroenterology (ACG) and Canadian Association of Gastroenterology (CAG) suggest that patients ≥60 years of age presenting with dyspepsia should undergo upper endoscopy to exclude any organic cause [40].

4. Management

4.1 Uncomplicated PUD

Risk factors for the development of PUD should be evaluated. Patients should be advised to avoid NSAID intake, stop smoking, and limit drinking of alcohol. If the patient is *H. pylori* positive, it should be treated, and eradication of infection should be confirmed ≥4 weeks after completion of therapy [37]. There are different

Regimen	Drugs	Duration	Eradication rate (%)
PAC therapy	PPI standard dose BID plus amoxicillin 1 g BID plus clarithromycin 500 mg BID	14 days	70–85
PAM therapy	PPI standard dose BID plus amoxicillin 1 g BID plus metronidazole 500 mg TID	14 days	70–85
Bismuth quadruple therapy	PPI standard dose BID plus bismuth subcitrate (120–300 mg) or subsalicylate (300 mg) QID plus tetracycline 500 mg QID plus metronidazole 250 MG QID	10–14 days	75–90
Concomitant therapy	PPI standard dose BID plus amoxicillin 1 g BID plus clarithromycin 500 mg BID plus metronidazole or tinidazole 500 mg BID	10–14 days	94.4
Sequential therapy	PPI standard dose plus amoxicillin 1 g BID for 5 days followed by PPI plus clarithromycin 500 mg plus either metronidazole or tinidazole 500 mg BID for additional 5 days	Total 10 days	84.4
Hybrid therapy	PPI standard dose plus amoxicillin 1 g BID for 7 days followed by PPI standard dose plus amoxicillin 1 g plus clarithromycin 500 mg plus metronidazole 500 mg BID for additional 7 days	Total 14 days	93.4
Levofloxacin triple therapy	PPI standard dose and amoxicillin 1 g BID plus levofloxacin 500 mg QD	10–14 days	83.1
Levofloxacin sequential therapy	PPI standard dose plus amoxicillin 1 g BID for 5–7 days followed by PPI standard dose plus amoxicillin 1 g plus metronidazole 500 mg BID and levofloxacin 500 mg QD for additional 5–7 days	Total 10–14 days	92.2
LOAD therapy	PPI (double dose) plus levofloxacin 250 mg plus doxycycline 100 mg QD and nitazoxanide 500 mg BID	7–10 days	88.9
Novel concomitant therapy	PPI standard dose and amoxicillin 1 g TID (if allergic to penicillin, bismuth subcitrate 240 mg QID) plus rifabutin 150 mg and ciprofloxacin 500 mg BID	10 days	Regimen with amoxicillin 95.2 Regimen with bismuth subcitrate 94.2

BID, twice a day; QID, four times a day; QD, once a day.

Table 1.
Treatment of H. pylori infection.

regimens of anti-*H. pylori* therapy available. Patients' previous history of antibiotic exposure and prevalence of regional antibiotic resistance should be taken into consideration. Treatment of *H. pylori* infection is summarized in **Table 1** [41]. Antibiotics, histamine 2 receptor antagonists (H2RA), PPI, sucralfate, and bismuth-containing medications (Pepto-Bismol) can interfere with the results of urea breath test and stool for *H. pylori* antigen test and may give a false-negative result. Patients should stop taking these medications at least 2 weeks prior to these tests [42, 43]. But patients can continue taking antacids (except Maalox total relief) as they do not affect the accuracy of the tests.

Bismuth quadruple therapy or concomitant therapy can be considered as the first-line therapy against *H. pylori* infection. PAC therapy should be considered as first-line treatment in patients without history of exposure to macrolide and living in an area where *H. pylori* clarithromycin resistance is low. If the first-line therapy fails, susceptibility testing should be done if available, and susceptibility-based therapy should be given. If susceptibility testing is not available, salvage therapy should not contain the antibiotics used before. For example, if bismuth quadruple therapy fails, clarithromycin- or levofloxacin-based therapy should be used as salvage therapy. If clarithromycin-based therapy fails, bismuth quadruple therapy or levofloxacin-based therapy should be used as salvage therapy. First-line therapy generally fails in 25% of cases as a result of non-compliance, antibiotic resistance, prior exposure to antibiotic, smoking, and younger age [44–46].

Acid suppressant therapy and mucosal cytoprotective agents are the main modes of therapy for the healing of PU. Acid suppressant therapy includes H2RAs and PPIs which are listed in **Tables 2** and **3**.

Duration of H2RA therapy: 90% of duodenal ulcers are healed by H2RA in 6–8 weeks, whereas 90% of gastric ulcers are healed by H2RA in 12 weeks [48].

Duration of PPI therapy: in the case of *H. pylori*-associated peptic ulcers, 90% of the ulcers are healed by a 2-week course of PPI plus antibiotics for eradication of *H. pylori* infection. This regimen followed by additional 2 weeks of PPI does not make much difference in healing of peptic ulcer. PPI therapy should be

H2RA	Dose	Side effects
Cimetidine	800 mg qhs × 4–8 weeks	Gynecomastia, impotence, polymyositis, interstitial nephritis, confusion, agitation, vitamin B12 deficiency
Ranitidine	150 mg BID × 4–8 weeks	Diarrhea, constipation, xerostomia, xeroderma Vitamin B12 deficiency
Famotidine	40 mg qhs × 4–8 weeks	Agranulocytosis, angioedema, anaphylaxis, seizure
Nizatidine	300 mg qhs × 4–8 weeks	Nausea, vomiting, dyspepsia, insomnia, somnolence, vitamin B12 deficiency

qhs, every night at bed time.

Table 2.
H2RA with dose and side effects.

PPI	Dose	Side effects
Omeprazole	20–40 mg qd × 4–8 weeks	Acute: headache, diarrhea
Esomeprazole	20–40 mg qd × 4–8 weeks	Chronic: hypocalcemia, hypomagnesemia, iron deficiency, vitamin B12 deficiency, *Clostridium difficile* infection, pneumonia, acute interstitial nephritis, risk of fracture, drug-induced lupus erythematosus [47]
Lansoprazole	15–30 mg qd × 4–8 weeks	
Dexlansoprazole	30–60 mg qd × 4–8 weeks	
Pantoprazole	20–40 mg qd × 4–8 weeks	
Rabeprazole	20 mg qd × 4–8 weeks	

qd, daily.

Table 3.
PPI with dose and side effects.

continued for 8 weeks in case of gastric ulcer and 4 weeks in case of duodenal ulcer [49].

In the case of NSAID-induced PUD, NSAIDs should be withdrawn if possible, but PPIs are the drugs of choice. PPIs should be continued for at least 8 weeks for the healing of PU. But maintenance dose of PPI should be continued to prevent ulcer complications if the patient needs to be on NSAID or aspirin for other medical conditions.

5. Mucosal cytoprotective agents

Misoprostol and sucralfate are mucosal cytoprotective agents.

Misoprostol is a synthetic analogue of prostaglandin E which is trophic to gastroduodenal mucosa, stimulates mucus and bicarbonate secretion from the gastroduodenal mucosa, and can form hydrophobic surfactant-like phospholipids in the gastric epithelial cells [50]. Misoprostol can also inhibit gastric acid secretion by suppressing histamine-stimulated cyclic AMP production but does not induce hypergastrinemia [51]. Misoprostol can heal both gastric and duodenal ulcers. Misoprostol 200 microgram four times a day should be given for 12 weeks. It can prevent mucosal damage and formation of ulcers from the deleterious effects of low-dose aspirin, NSAIDs, smoking, and alcohol [52]. Misoprostol is approved in the United States for the prevention of NSAID-induced PUD. As misoprostol can accelerate intestinal transit time and increase intestinal water and electrolyte secretion, abdominal cramps and mild to moderate diarrhea can happen in up to 30% of cases. Diarrhea can be reduced by taking food with misoprostol. Misoprostol can also cause nausea, vomiting, menstrual cramps, and vaginal bleeding (due to uterine contraction). Misoprostol is contraindicated in pregnant patients.

Sucralfate is the aluminum salt of sulfated sucrose. It coats the gastroduodenal mucosa (both ulcerated and non-ulcerated areas); binds acid and pepsin; stimulates the secretion of bicarbonate, prostaglandin, and epidermal growth factor; and thus helps in healing of PU. Sucralfate is as good as H2RA in healing PU (duodenal ulcer 60–90% at 4–6 weeks and gastric ulcer 90% at 12 weeks) and has a lower rate of recurrence of duodenal ulcer after healing as compared to H2RA [53, 54]. In the United States, sucralfate is approved for the treatment of active duodenal ulcer not related to NSAID. Side effects of sucralfate include nausea, vomiting, gastric upset, itching, and skin rash. Less than 5% of sucralfate is absorbed from the gastrointestinal tract into the systemic circulation and eliminated primarily in the urine. Sucralfate should be avoided in patients with chronic kidney disease as it contains aluminum.

6. Role of follow-up endoscopy

In the case of gastric ulcer, follow-up endoscopy is recommended 12 weeks after medical therapy to evaluate for underlying malignancy. Surveillance endoscopy should be individualized:

1. Surveillance endoscopy is necessary in patients with giant ulcer (>2 cm) and malignant-looking ulcer (thick mucosal folds, irregular ulcer edges, mass lesion) on index endoscopy; ulcer biopsy was not done on initial endoscopy; initial endoscopy was done for upper gastrointestinal bleeding and unknown etiology of the ulcer; patient remains symptomatic even after taking medical therapy; index endoscopy showed gastric atrophy, intestinal metaplasia,

dysplasia, or adenoma; and patient has risk factors for gastric cancer which include *H. pylori* positivity, age > 50 years, family history of gastric cancer, and coming from a high prevalent area of gastric cancer (South Korea, Mongolia, Japan, China, Bhutan, Kyrgyzstan, Chile, etc.). If the gastric ulcer seems to be active or healing on surveillance endoscopy, four-quadrant biopsies from the edges and base of the ulcer should be taken [55].

2. Surveillance endoscopy may not be necessary if the patient does not have any risk factor for malignancy and the gastric ulcer is small, benign appearing, and antral in location due to NSAID and the initial biopsy does not show any dysplasia or malignancy [56].

In case of duodenal ulcer, surveillance endoscopy is generally not required because of low risk of malignancy. But if the patient remains symptomatic or symptoms recur despite medical therapy, surveillance endoscopy should be considered to evaluate for refractory ulcer or non-peptic nature of the ulcer which includes Crohn's disease, lymphoma, or tuberculosis.

7. Refractory and recurrent ulcers

When the ulcer does not heal up after a 12-week course of PPI therapy, it is called refractory ulcer. 5–10% ulcers are refractory ulcers. When the ulcer recurs after complete healing of the ulcer, it is called recurrent ulcer. 5–30% ulcers are recurrent ulcers. The two most important causes of refractory and recurrent ulcers are continued NSAID use and persistent *H. pylori* infection [57]. Other important factors include cigarette smoking, smoking of crack cocaine, concurrent use of corticosteroid, cytotoxic drugs (sirolimus, mycophenolate mofetil), alendronate, methamphetamine, idiopathic hypersecretory duodenal ulcer, antral G-cell hyperplasia, gastrinoma, Crohn's disease, sarcoidosis, cancer, non-*H. pylori* infection (*Helicobacter heilmannii*), and infiltrative condition like gastrointestinal stromal tumor and Kaposi sarcoma.

Patients with refractory or recurrent ulcers should be thoroughly investigated to find out the causative factors which should be addressed. Twice daily PPI therapy should be given for another 12 weeks. Then upper endoscopy should be done to document complete healing of the ulcer. Patients with gastric ulcer should be referred for surgery if ulcer does not heal by 24 weeks.

8. Complications

Common complications of PUD include bleeding, perforation, penetration, and gastric outlet obstruction.

8.1 Bleeding

About 50% of all cases of upper gastrointestinal bleeding are caused by PUD [58]. Patients may present with hematemesis, melena, anemia, or heme-positive stool. At presentation, the patient's hemodynamic status (pulse, blood pressure) should be checked and resuscitative measures should be started. Patients should be given intravenous crystalloid fluid to maintain blood pressure, and parenteral PPI (esomeprazole or pantoprazole) should be started (continuous infusion or twice daily intravenously). PPI therapy increases intragastric pH with stabilization of blood clot and reduces the risk of rebleeding and the need for surgery but does not decrease overall mortality [59]. Blood transfusion should be given to keep the hemoglobin ≥7 gm/dl, but in patients with hypovolemia or comorbidities like coronary artery disease, hemoglobin target should be higher. Risk assessment should be done to categorize high-risk or low-risk patients, level of care, need for blood transfusion, timing of endoscopy, and timing of discharge. The Glasgow-Blatchford bleeding score (GBS) is a useful screening tool (**Table 4**) to determine the need for intervention [60]. Patients with a score of 0 are considered as low risk with minimum risk of needing interventions like blood transfusion, endoscopy, and surgery, and they should be considered for early discharge from the hospital. But all other values (>0) fall into the category of high risk in terms of need for blood transfusion, endoscopy, and surgery. A score of 6 or more has >50% risk of needing intervention.

After resuscitation and stabilization, EGD should be done for diagnostic and therapeutic purposes. During endoscopy, Forrest classification should be used to assess the need for endoscopic intervention [61]. The different Forrest classes with their prevalence and risk of rebleeding are mentioned in **Table 5** [62]. Patients with Forrest classes Ia, Ib, IIa, and IIb are considered to be high-risk candidates, and endoscopic treatment should be provided to reduce the risk of rebleeding. Patients with Forrest classes IIc and III do not require any endoscopic intervention. In fact,

Admission risk marker	Score component value
Blood urea (mmol/L)	
6.5–8.0	2
8.0–10.0	3
10.0–25	4
>25	6
Hemoglobin (g/dL) for men	
12.0–12.9	1
10.0–11.9	3
<10.0	6
Hemoglobin (g/dL) for women	
10.0–11.9	1
<10.0	6
Systolic blood pressure (mm Hg)	
100–109	1
90–99	2
<90	3
Other markers	
Pulse ≥100 (per min)	1
Presentation with melena	1
Presentation with syncope	2
Hepatic disease	2
Cardiac failure	2

Table 4.
GBS.

Forrest class	Endoscopic finding	Prevalence (%)	Risk of recurrent bleeding on medical management (%)
Ia	Spurting arterial bleed	10	90
Ib	Oozing of blood without visible vessel	10	10–20
IIa	Non-bleeding visible vessel	25	50
IIb	Adherent blood clot	10	25–30
IIc	Flat pigmented spot	10	7–10
III	Clean-based ulcer	35	3–5

Table 5.
Forrest classes with prevalence and risk of recurrent bleeding.

patients with Forrest class III can resume a regular diet and can be discharged home as long as they are hemodynamically stable, with stable hemoglobin and without other comorbidities, and they have somebody at home to watch them [63].

Endoscopic treatment options can categorized into three main types:

1. *Injection therapy*: it is the oldest endoscopic hemostatic method. Epinephrine (1:10,000 dilution) 0.2–2 ml aliquots are injected in four quadrants of the bleeding stigmata. Initial hemostasis is obtained by its tamponade effect as well as vasoconstrictive effect. But as it is less effective as a monotherapy, other modalities of endoscopic treatment are added for better hemostasis [64].

2. *Thermal therapy*: it includes contact methods by bipolar or monopolar cauterization and noncontact method by argon plasma coagulation (APC). Contact methods work by coaptive coagulation. Bipolar cauterization is most commonly used nowadays. A combination of epinephrine injection and bipolar cauterization is more effective than either modality alone in achieving hemostasis [65]. The APC machine has a high-frequency monopolar electrosurgical generator, argon gas chamber, gas flowmeter, grounding pad, flexible APC delivery catheter, and foot switch to activate gas and energy. Argon gas release with delivery of electric current is synchronized by the foot switch. The APC probe should be within 2–8 mm from the site of the targeted tissue to induce plasma coagulation. The depth of the burn can be preset between 0.5 and 3 mm. APC is an effective method of hemostasis in bleeding peptic ulcer [66]. But APC can cause superficial ulcerations which are generally healed up in 2–3 weeks.

3. *Mechanical therapy*: endoclips are widely used to stop bleeding from peptic ulcer. There are different clips available which include resolution clip, endoscopic hemoclip, Quick Clip2 (rotatable clip), Duraclip, and SureClip. All these clips can go through the standard 2.8 mm endoscope channel and can stop bleeding by grasping the bleeding vessel, reducing the chance of rebleeding and need for surgery. Endoclips have been found to be superior to injection therapy but comparable to thermocoagulation in bleeding PU [67]. They do not cause any tissue trauma, and as a result, ulcer healing is not impaired. They are also MRI compatible. Disadvantages of endoclipping include the following: (a) sometimes technical difficulty to clip the lesions in locations like the posterior duodenal bulb, posterior gastric body, and proximal lesser curve of the stomach, (b) limitation of use in large blood vessel (>2 mm

in diameter), (c) difficulty to grasp fibrotic tissue, and (d) requirement of multiple clips [68].

Another clip called Ovesco clip is an over-the-scope clip used to stop peptic ulcer bleeding. The bleeding area is suctioned into a cup attached to the scope, and then the clip is deployed like band ligation.

A combination of at least two modalities of endoscopic treatment (injection, thermal, or mechanical) is now the standard of care in the treatment of peptic ulcer bleeding.

9. Endoscopic Doppler ultrasound

An ultrasound probe is passed through the endoscope channel and placed directly onto the area of bleeding. An audible sound is heard if there is blood flow. Arterial or venous blood flow can be detected. It is useful after endoscopic treatment to evaluate the presence of any residual blood flow which can increase the potential for rebleeding. It is also useful in Forrest IIc and III ulcers to find out any vascular signal. Doppler ultrasound-guided endoscopic hemostasis reduces 30-day rebleeding rate significantly and is also cost-effective [69].

Hemospray or hemostatic nanopowder is an alternative approach to obtain hemostasis. The powder is delivered through a catheter which passes through the endoscope channel, and the powder is then sprayed over the bleeding site. The powder forms a stable mechanical barrier at the site of bleeding. Initial success rate in obtaining hemostasis is 75–100%, but rebleeding rate is 10–49% [70]. So hemospray should be used as a bridge therapy in massive peptic ulcer bleeding when standard endoscopic treatment fails.

Endoscopic therapy can control acute peptic ulcer bleeding with high success. Primary hemostasis can be obtained in more than 90% of cases, but rebleeding can occur in up to 15% of cases after therapeutic endoscopic procedure [71].

10. Role of second-look endoscopy

Second-look endoscopy is not routinely recommended after initial endoscopy for the management of PU bleeding unless the endoscopist is concerned that suboptimal treatment was given in the first endoscopy or there was poor visualization due to blood or food debris during the first endoscopy [72].

11. Complications of endoscopic treatment

Complications could be due to sedation, patients' comorbidities, and endoscopy itself. Sedation-related complications include hypoventilation, hypoxia, aspiration pneumonia, airway obstruction, arrhythmia, pulmonary embolism, myocardial infarction, phlebitis, and vasovagal attack [73]. The complications of endoscopic hemostasis include exacerbation of bleeding and perforation, but the overall incidence is $<0.5\%$. The rate of perforation after contact thermal therapy could be as high as 2%. Following thermal therapy, induction or exacerbation of bleeding can occur in up to 5% of cases [74].

12. Failure of endoscopic therapy

If the endoscopic therapy fails to achieve hemostasis, the next step will be angiography with transarterial embolization (TAE). Different agents are used for embolization, and these include Gelfoam, endocoils, cyanoacrylic glues, and polyvinyl alcohol. The success rate of TAE in obtaining hemostasis is 52–98%, but recurrent bleeding can occur in 10–20%, requiring repeat TAE [75].

13. Role of surgery

Surgery is indicated if TAE fails to stop PU bleeding. Emergency surgery involves plication or oversewing of the ulcer with ligation of the bleeding artery and truncal vagotomy and pyloroplasty. Wong et al. compared surgery vs. TAE in bleeding PU patients who had failed endoscopic therapy. Surgery was associated with less recurrent bleeding but more complications when compared with TAE. There was no significant difference in the mean length of hospital stay, need for blood transfusion, and 30-day mortality between the two groups [76]. In practice, the surgical intervention continues to diminish, but the radiological intervention continues to increase in acute PU bleeding patients who have unsuccessful endoscopic therapy. Surgery is also recommended for (a) patients with perforation, (b) shock due to recurrent bleeding, (c) patients with hemodynamic instability despite adequate resuscitative measures needing more than three units of blood transfusion, and (d) unavailability of interventional radiology.

14. Prognosis of bleeding peptic ulcer

The outcome depends on successful endoscopic hemostasis without recurrent bleeding. The risk factors for recurrent bleeding include patients with renal failure on dialysis; elderly patients on NSAID, antiplatelet agents, and anticoagulants; patients with ulcer located on the posterior duodenal wall and lesser curve of the stomach; and patients with active bleeding ulcer during endoscopy. Despite the tremendous advances in technology, the mortality of acute PU bleeding remains about 10% [77].

15. Perforation

In patients with PUD, the lifetime prevalence of perforation is 5%. Patients generally present with acute abdomen. The triad of sudden onset of abdominal pain, tachycardia, and abdominal rigidity is highly suggestive of PU perforation. Smoking, NSAIDs, corticosteroids, old age, *H. pylori* infection, stress, and previous history of PUD are risk factors for perforation [78]. Upright chest X-ray is generally diagnostic, but it can miss free air under the diaphragm in 15% of cases. CT (computerized tomography) is very sensitive in detecting the presence and site of perforation [79]. CT with oral contrast may also show leak. Exploratory laparotomy with omental patch is the treatment of choice. PU perforation carries increased risk of morbidity and mortality if not treated early.

16. Penetration

When the ulcer crater erodes through the gastric wall or intestinal wall into the surrounding structure but there is no free perforation or leakage of luminal contents into the peritoneal cavity, it is called penetration [80]. The pancreas is the commonest site of penetration. Other sites of penetration include the omentum, biliary tract, liver, colon, mesocolon, and blood vessels. Patients may notice change in pattern of abdominal pain, i.e., pain not being relieved by taking food or medication. Diagnosis is confirmed by CT with contrast which may show loss of fascial plane between the gastric wall or intestinal wall and the surrounding structure, band of soft tissue density between them, ulcer crater, sinus tract, and enlargement of head of the pancreas in case of penetration into the pancreas [81]. Treatment is surgical intervention.

17. Gastric outlet obstruction (GOO)

It occurs in less than 5% cases of PUD. Duodenal ulcer and pyloric channel ulcer are generally associated with GOO. Pathophysiologically, reversible causes like inflammation, edema, spasm, and pyloric dysmotility and irreversible cause like fibrosis may lead to GOO. Patients present with nausea, vomiting, early satiety, epigastric pain, and weight loss. Patients may develop severe dehydration, azotemia, hyponatremia, and hypochloremic and hypokalemic metabolic alkalosis with paradoxical aciduria due to prolonged vomiting. First, the fluid and electrolyte deficit should be corrected. Gastric contents should be removed by large-bore Ewald tube, and then intermittent nasogastric tube suction should be continued for a few days. Many cases of GOO due to PUD have reversible components which may respond to this conservative treatment. Patients not responding to the conservative treatment need endoscopic dilation or surgery [82, 83].

18. Conclusion

PUD is a common clinical problem. The two most important risk factors are *H. pylori* infection and NSAIDs. Patients may present with dyspepsia or may remain asymptomatic. Endoscopy is the gold standard for the diagnosis of PUD. But as it is not possible to endoscope so many dyspeptic patients, there are some non-endoscopic approaches depending on the prevalence of *H. pylori* infection in the population. But ACG and CAG recommend EGD to be done in patients ≥60 years of age presenting with dyspepsia irrespective of alarm features. Bismuth quadruple therapy or concomitant therapy should be considered as the first-line therapy against *H. pylori* infection. In patients with PUD, eradication of *H. pylori* infection (if positive) should be confirmed ≥4 weeks after completion of therapy. PPI, H2RA, misoprostol, and sucralfate are the main agents used for healing of PU. Surveillance endoscopy is recommended in certain gastric ulcers. PUD can be complicated by bleeding, perforation, penetration, and gastric outlet obstruction. Patients with bleeding peptic ulcer should be evaluated, resuscitated, and started on intravenous/infusion of PPI. Diagnostic and therapeutic endoscopy should be done to achieve endoscopic hemostasis. If endoscopic therapy fails, the next step will be TAE or surgery. The mortality for peptic ulcer bleeding still remains high.

Author details

Monjur Ahmed
Jefferson University Hospital, Philadelphia, USA

*Address all correspondence to: monjur.ahmed@jefferson.edu

References

[1] Lanas A, Chan FKL. Peptic ulcer disease. Lancet. 2017;**390**(10094):613-624

[2] Yuan Y, Leontiadis GI. Ulcer-related vs non-ulcer-nonvariceal upper gastrointestinal bleeding-which has worse outcomes? Alimentary Pharmacology and Therapeutics. 2019;**49**(6):818-819

[3] Adam V, Barkun AN. Estimates of costs of hospital stay for variceal and nonvariceal upper gastrointestinal bleeding in the United States. Value in Health. 2008;**11**(1):1-3

[4] Sandler RS, Everhart JE, Donowitz M, Adams E, Cronin K, Goodman C, et al. The burden of selected digestive diseases in the United States. Gastroenterology. 2002;**122**(5):1500-1501

[5] Everhart JE, Kruszon-Moran D, Perez-Perez GI, Tralka TS, McQuillan G. Seroprevalence and ethnic differences in *Helicobacter pylori* infection among adults in the United States. Journal of Infectious Diseases. 2000;**181**(4):1359-1363

[6] Salih BA. *Helicobacter pylori* infection in developing countries: The burden for how long? Saudi Journal of Gastroenterology. 2009;**15**(3):201-207

[7] Sung JJ, Kuipers EJ, El-Serag HB. Systematic review: The global incidence and prevalence of peptic ulcer disease. Alimentary Pharmacology and Therapeutics. 2009;**29**(9):938-946

[8] O'Connor HJ. The role of *Helicobacter pylori* in peptic ulcer disease. Scandinavian Journal of Gastroenterology. Supplement. 1994;**201**:11-15

[9] Uyanikoğlu A, Danalioğlu A, Akyüz F, Ermış F, Güllüoğlu M, Kapran Y, et al. Etiological factors of duodenal and gastric ulcers. Turkish Journal of Gastroenterology. 2012;**23**(2):99-103

[10] Kawamura N, Ito Y, Sasaki M, Iida A, Mizuno M, Ogasawara N, et al. Low-dose aspirin-associated upper gastric and duodenal ulcers in Japanese patients with no previous history of peptic ulcers. BMC Research Notes. 2013;**6**:455

[11] Silen W. What is cytoprotection of gastric mucosa? Gastroenterology. 1988;**94**(1):232-234

[12] Drini M. Peptic ulcer disease and non-steroidal anti-inflammatory drugs. Australian Prescriber. 2017;**40**(3):91-93

[13] Laine L. Approaches to nonsteroidal anti-inflammatory drug use in the high-risk patient. Gastroenterology. 2001;**120**:594-606

[14] Abu-Taleb AMF, Abdelattef RS, Abdel-Hady AA, Omran FH, El-Korashi LA, Abdel-Aziz El-Hady H, et al. Prevalence of *Helicobacter pylori* cagA and iceA genes and their association with gastrointestinal diseases. International Journal of Microbiology. 2018;**2018**:4809093

[15] Suzuki R, Shiota S, Yamaoka Y. Molecular epidemiology, population genetics, and pathogenic role of *Helicobacter pylori*. Infection, Genetics and Evolution. 2012;**12**(2):203-213

[16] Foegeding NJ, Caston RR, McClain MS, Ohi MD, Cover TL. An overview of *Helicobacter pylori* VacA toxin biology. Toxins (Basel). 2016;**8**(6):pii: E173

[17] Calam J. *Helicobacter pylori* and somatostatin cells. European Journal of Gastroenterology and Hepatology. 1998;**10**(4):281-283

[18] Futami H, Takashima M, Furuta T, Hanai H, Kaneko E. Relationship

between *Helicobacter pylori* infection and gastric metaplasia in the duodenal bulb in the pathogenesis of duodenal ulcer. Journal of Gastroenterology and Hepatology. 1999;**14**(2):114-119

[19] Mertz HR, Walsh JH. Peptic ulcer pathophysiology. Medical Clinics of North America. 1991;**75**(4):799-814

[20] Available from: https://emedicine.medscape.com/article/184332-overview

[21] Hirasuna JD, Shelub I, Bolt RJ. Hyperhistaminemia and peptic ulcer. Western Journal of Medicine. 1979;**131**(2):140-143

[22] Dall M, Schaffalitzky de Muckadell OB, Lassen AT, Hallas J. There is an association between selective serotonin reuptake inhibitor use and uncomplicated peptic ulcers: A population-based case-control study. Alimentary Pharmacology and Therapeutics. 2010;**32**(11–12):1383-1391

[23] Debongnie JC, Donnay M, Mairesse J, Lamy V, Dekoninck X, Ramdani B. Gastric ulcers and *Helicobacter heilmannii*. European Journal of Gastroenterology and Hepatology. 1998;**10**(3):251-254

[24] Stemboroski L, Gaye B, Makary R, Monteiro C, Eid E. Isolated gastrointestinal sarcoidosis involving multiple gastrointestinal sites presenting as chronic diarrhea. ACG Case Reports Journal. 2016;**3**(4):e198

[25] Schlemper RJ, van der Werf SD, Vandenbroucke JP, Biemond I, Lamers CB. Risk factors of peptic ulcer disease: Different impact of *Helicobacter pylori* in Dutch and Japanese populations? Journal of Gastroenterology and Hepatology. 1996;**11**(9):825-831 8889960

[26] Jaff MS. Relation between ABO blood groups and *Helicobacter pylori* infection in symptomatic patients. Clinical and Experimental Gastroenterology. 2011;**4**:221-226

[27] Lambert R, Martin F. Susceptibility to peptic ulcer and blood group substances. Digestion. 1969;**2**:298-303

[28] Ansari SA, Khan A, Khan TA, Raza Y, Syed SA, Akhtar SS, et al. Correlation of ABH blood group antigens secretion with *Helicobacter pylori* infection in Pakistani patients. Tropical Medicine and International Health. 2015;**20**(1): 115-119

[29] Malaty HM, Graham DY, Isaksson I, Engstrand L, Pedersen NL. Are genetic influences on peptic ulcer dependent or independent of genetic influences for *Helicobacter pylori* infection? Archives of Internal Medicine. 2000;**160**(1):105-109

[30] Jones MP. The role of psychosocial factors in peptic ulcer disease: Beyond *Helicobacter pylori* and NSAIDs. Journal of Psychosomatic Research. 2006;**60**(4): 407-412

[31] Anand BS. Peptic Ulcer Disease Clinical Presentation. Available from: https://emedicine.medscape.com/article/181753-clinical

[32] Hilton D, Iman N, Burke GJ, Moore A, O'Mara G, Signorini D, et al. Absence of abdominal pain in older persons with endoscopic ulcers: A prospective study. The American Journal of Gastroenterology. 2001;**96**(2):380-384

[33] Matthewson K, Pugh S, Northfield TC. Which peptic ulcer patients bleed? Gut. 1988;**29**(1):70-74

[34] Ramakrisnan K, Salinas RC. Peptic ulcer disease. American Family Physician. 2007;**76**(7):1005-1012

[35] Lash JG, Genta RM. Adherence to the Sydney system guidelines increases the detection of *Helicobacter gastritis* and intestinal metaplasia in 400738 sets of gastric biopsies. Alimentary

Pharmacology and Therapeutics. 2013; **38**(4):424-431

[36] Loyd RA, McClellan DA. Update on the evaluation and management of functional dyspepsia. American Family Physician. 2011;**83**(5):547-552

[37] Malfertheiner P, Megraud F, O'Morain CA, Gisbert JP, Kuipers EJ, Axon AT, et al. European Helicobacter and Microbiota study group and consensus panel. Management of *Helicobacter pylori* infection-the Maastricht V/Florence consensus report. Gut. 2017;**66**(1):6-30

[38] Talley NJ, American Gastroenterological Association. American Gastroenterological Association medical position statement: Evaluation of dyspepsia. Gastroenterology. 2005;**129**(5): 1753-1755

[39] Talley NJ, Vakil N, Practice Parameters Committee of the American College of Gastroenterology. Guidelines for the management of dyspepsia. The American Journal of Gastroenterology. 2005;**100**(10):2324-2337

[40] Moayyedi PM, Lacy BE, Andrews CN, Enns RA, Howden CW, Vakil N. ACG and CAG clinical guideline: Management of dyspepsia. American Journal of Gastroenterology. 2017; **112**(7):988-1013

[41] Chey WD, Leontiadis GI, Howden CW, Moss SF. ACG clinical guideline: Treatment of *Helicobacter pylori* infection. The American Journal of Gastroenterology. 2017;**112**(2): 212-239

[42] Bravo LE, Realpe JL, Campo C, Mera R, Correa P. Effects of acid suppression and bismuth medications on the performance of diagnostic tests for *Helicobacter pylori* infection. The American Journal of Gastroenterology. 1999;**94**(9):2380-2383

[43] Lee HJ, Kim JI, Lee JS, Jun EJ, Oh JH, Cheung DY, et al. Concomitant therapy achieved the best eradication rate for *Helicobacter pylori* among various treatment strategies. World Journal of Gastroenterology. 2015;**21**(1): 351-359

[44] Megraud F, Coenen S, Versporten A, Kist M, Lopez-Brea M, Hirschl AM, et al. *Helicobacter pylori* resistance to antibiotics in Europe and its relationship to antibiotic consumption. Gut. 2013; **62**(1):34-42

[45] Broutet N, Tchamgoué S, Pereira E, Lamouliatte H, Salamon R, Mégraud F. Risk factors for failure of *Helicobacter pylori* therapy—Results of an individual data analysis of 2751 patients. Alimentary Pharmacology and Therapeutics. 2003;**17**(1):99-109

[46] Suzuki T, Matsuo K, Ito H, Sawaki A, Hirose K, Wakai K, et al. Smoking increases the treatment failure for *Helicobacter pylori* eradication. The American Journal of Medicine. 2006; **119**(3):217-224

[47] Sandholdt LH, Laurinaviciene R, Bygum A. Proton pump inhibitor-induced subacute cutaneous lupus erythematosus. British Journal of Dermatology. 2014;**170**(2):342-351

[48] Rubin W. Medical treatment of peptic ulcer disease. Medical Clinics of North America. 1991;**75**(4):981-998

[49] Gisbert JP, Pajares JM. Systematic review and meta-analysis: Is 1-week proton pump inhibitor-based triple therapy sufficient to heal peptic ulcer? Alimentary Pharmacology and Therapeutics. 2005;**21**:795-804

[50] Aly A. Prostaglandins in clinical treatment of gastroduodenal mucosal lesions: A review. Scandinavian Journal of Gastroenterology. Supplement. 1987; **137**:43-49

[51] Watkinson G, Hopkins A, Akbar FA. The therapeutic efficacy of misoprostol in peptic ulcer disease. Postgraduate Medical Journal. 1988;**64**(Suppl 1):60-77

[52] Wilson DE. Misoprostol and gastroduodenal mucosal protection (cytoprotection). Postgraduate Medical Journal. 1988;**64**(Suppl 1):7-11

[53] Jensen SL, Funch Jensen P. Role of sucralfate in peptic disease. Digestive Diseases. 1992;**10**(3):153-161

[54] Hunt RH. Treatment of peptic ulcer disease with sucralfate: A review. The American Journal of Medicine. 1991;**91**(2A):102S-106S

[55] Lv SX, Gan JH, Wang CC, Luo EP, Huang XP, Xie Y, et al. Biopsy from the base of gastric ulcer may find gastric cancer earlier. Medical Hypotheses. 2011;**76**(2):249-250

[56] Gielisse EA, Kuyvenhoven JP. Follow-up endoscopy for benign-appearing gastric ulcers has no additive value in detecting malignancy: It is time to individualise surveillance endoscopy. Gastric Cancer. 2015;**18**(4):803-809

[57] Kim HU. Diagnostic and treatment approaches for refractory peptic ulcers. Clinical Endoscopy. 2015;**48**(4):285-290

[58] Arlt GD, Leyh M. Incidence and pathophysiology of peptic ulcer bleeding. Langenbeck's Archives of Surgery. 2001;**386**(2):75-81

[59] Leontiadis GI, Sharma VK, Howden CW. Systematic review and meta-analysis of proton pump inhibitor therapy in peptic ulcer bleeding. BMJ. 2005;**330**(7491):568

[60] Blatchford O, Murray WR, Blatchford M. A risk score to predict need for treatment for upper-gastrointestinal haemorrhage. Lancet. 2000;**356**(9238):1318-1321

[61] Forrest JA, Finlayson ND, Shearman DJ. Endoscopy in gastrointestinal bleeding. Lancet. 1974;**2**(7877):394-397

[62] Katschinski B, Logan R, Davies J, Faulkner G, Pearson J, Langman M. Prognostic factors in upper gastrointestinal bleeding. Digestive Diseases and Sciences. 1994;**39**(4): 706-712

[63] Laine L, Jensen DM. Management of patients with ulcer bleeding. The American Journal of Gastroenterology. 2012;**107**(3):345-360

[64] Kim JS, Park SM, Kim BW. Endoscopic management of peptic ulcer bleeding. Clinical Endoscopy. 2015; **48**(2):106-111

[65] Bianco MA, Rotondano G, Marmo R, Piscopo R, Orsini L, Cipolletta L. Combined epinephrine and bipolar probe coagulation vs. bipolar probe coagulation alone for bleeding peptic ulcer: A randomized, controlled trial. Gastrointestinal Endoscopy. 2004; **60**(6):910-915

[66] Karaman A, Baskol M, Gursoy S, Torun E, Yurci A, Ozel BD, et al. Epinephrine plus argon plasma or heater probe coagulation in ulcer bleeding. World Journal of Gastroenterology. 2011;**17**(36):4109-4112

[67] Sung JJ, Tsoi KK, Lai LH, Wu JC, Lau JY. Endoscopic clipping versus injection and thermo-coagulation in the treatment of non-variceal upper gastrointestinal bleeding: A meta-analysis. Gut. 2007;**56**(10):1364-1373

[68] Technology Assessment Committee, Chuttani R, Barkun A, Carpenter S, Chotiprasidhi P, Ginsberg GG, et al. Endoscopic clip application devices. Gastrointestinal Endoscopy. 2006; **63**(6):746-750

[69] Jensen DM, Kovacs TOG, Ohning GV, Ghassemi K, Machicado GA, Dulai

GS, et al. Doppler endoscopic probe monitoring of blood flow improves risk stratification and outcomes of patients with severe nonvariceal upper gastrointestinal hemorrhage. Gastroenterology. 2017;**152**(6):1310-1318

[70] Yau AH, Ou G, Galorport C, Amar J, Bressler B, Donnellan F, et al. Safety and efficacy of Hemospray® in upper gastrointestinal bleeding. Canadian Journal of Gastroenterology and Hepatology. 2014;**28**(2):72-76

[71] Wong SH, Sung JJ. Management of patients with rebleeding. Gastrointestinal Endoscopy Clinics of North America. 2015;**25**(3):569-581

[72] Barkun AN, Bardou M, Kuipers EJ, Sung J, Hunt RH, Martel M, et al. International consensus recommendations on the management of patients with nonvariceal upper gastrointestinal bleeding. Annals of Internal Medicine. 2010;**152**(2):101-113

[73] Sharma VK, Nguyen CC, Crowell MD, Lieberman DA, de Garmo P, Fleischer DE. A national study of cardiopulmonary unplanned events after GI endoscopy. Gastrointestinal Endoscopy. 2007;**66**(1):27-34

[74] ASGE Standards of Practice Committee, Ben-Menachem T, Decker GA, Early DS, Evans J, Fanelli RD, et al. Adverse events of upper GI endoscopy. Gastrointestinal Endoscopy. 2012;**76**(4):707-718

[75] Gralnek IM. Will surgery be a thing of the past in peptic ulcer bleeding? Gastrointestinal Endoscopy. 2011;**73**(5):909-910

[76] Wong TC, Wong KT, Chiu PW, Teoh AY, Yu SC, Au KW, et al. A comparison of angiographic embolization with surgery after failed endoscopic hemostasis to bleeding peptic ulcers. Gastrointestinal Endoscopy. 2011;**73**(5):900-908

[77] Lau JY, Barkun A, Fan DM, Kuipers EJ, Yang YS, Chan FK. Challenges in the management of acute peptic ulcer bleeding. Lancet. 2013;**381**(9882):2033-2043

[78] Chung KT, Shelat VG. Perforated peptic ulcer—An update. World Journal of Gastrointestinal Surgery. 2017;**9**(1):1-12

[79] Hainaux B, Agneessens E, Bertinotti R, De Maertelaer V, Rubesova E, Capelluto E, et al. Accuracy of MDCT in predicting site of gastrointestinal tract perforation. AJR. American Journal of Roentgenology. 2006;**187**(5):1179-1183

[80] Pasumarthy L, Kumar RR, Srour J, Ahlbrandt D. Penetration of gastric ulcer into the splenic artery: A rare complication. Gastroenterology Research. 2009;**2**(6):350-352

[81] Madrazo BL, Halpert RD, Sandler MA, Pearlberg JL. Computed tomographic findings in penetrating peptic ulcer. Radiology. 1984;**153**(3):751-754

[82] DiSario JA, Fennerty MB, Tietze CC, Hutson WR, Burt RW. Endoscopic balloon dilation for ulcer-induced gastric outlet obstruction. The American Journal of Gastroenterology. 1994;**89**(6):868-871

[83] Weiland D, Dunn DH, Humphrey EW, Schwartz ML. Gastric outlet obstruction in peptic ulcer disease: An indication for surgery. The American Journal of Surgery. 1982;**143**(1):90-93

Chapter 2

Mid-Gastrointestinal Bleeding

Monjur Ahmed

Abstract

Mid-gastrointestinal bleeding constitutes a small proportion of all cases of gastrointestinal bleeding. It is more difficult to manage mid-gastrointestinal bleeding than upper or lower gastrointestinal bleeding. The etiology differs in younger and older age groups. The clinical presentation, investigations, and management are also different. Capsule endoscopy has improved the diagnostic accuracy to a great extent. Device-assisted enteroscopies (balloon-assisted enteroscopies and spiral enteroscopy) have both diagnostic and therapeutic potentials. Most of the time, patients present with obscure gastrointestinal bleeding which could be overt or occult. Another common presentation is iron deficiency anemia. A stepwise approach is essential to accurately diagnose and manage mid-gastrointestinal bleeding.

Keywords: small bowel bleed, occult gastrointestinal bleed, obscure gastrointestinal bleed, capsule endoscopy and gastrointestinal bleed, small bowel angioectasia

1. Introduction

Most of the gastrointestinal (GI) bleeding occurs from the upper and lower gastrointestinal tract. Mid-gastrointestinal (GI) bleeding refers to small bowel bleed anywhere from the ampulla of Vater to the ileocecal valve [1]. It occurs in 5–10% of all cases of gastrointestinal bleeding [2]. It is the most common cause of obscure GI bleeding, i.e., when the source of bleeding cannot be identified anywhere in the gastrointestinal tract [3, 4]. Management of mid-GI bleeding can be challenging to a gastroenterologist although various diagnostic and therapeutic tools are now available to evaluate and treat mid-GI bleeding. Despite the availability of various endoscopies and imaging studies, the exact cause of mid-GI bleeding can be still elusive in about one third of cases [5]. The etiology, clinical presentation, evaluation, investigations, and management of mid-GI bleeding will be discussed in this chapter.

2. Etiology

There are various etiologies of mid-GI bleeding, but their frequency depends on patient's age and underlying comorbidities [6]. Below the age of 40, the most common causes include Crohn's disease, Dieulafoy's lesion, small bowel tumors, Meckel's diverticulum, and polyposis syndrome. Small bowel tumors could be benign or malignant [7]. Benign ones include small gastrointestinal stromal tumors (GIST), benign neuroendocrine tumors (particularly small carcinoid), hemangioma, adenoma, leiomyoma, lipoma, and neurofibroma. Malignant ones include large GIST, adenocarcinoma, lymphoma, malignant neuroendocrine tumors, leiomyosarcoma, and metastatic tumor from melanoma, lung, or breast [8–11].

Rarely, polyposis syndromes involving the small bowel may present with mid-GI bleeding. These include familial adenomatous polyposis, Peutz-Jeghers syndrome, and generalized juvenile polyposis. Over the age of 40, the most common causes of mid-GI bleeding include angioectasia, nonsteroidal anti-inflammatory drug (NSAID)-induced ulcers, Dieulafoy's lesion, and small bowel tumors. On rare occasions, other small bowel lesions can cause gastrointestinal bleeding. These include small intestinal diverticuli, small intestinal varices, hereditary hemorrhagic telangiectasia, Kaposi sarcoma, intestinal tuberculosis, blue rubber bleb nevus syndrome, hematobilia, hemosuccus entericus, aortoenteric fistula, infectious enteritis, radiation enteritis, ulcerative jejunoileitis due to celiac disease, cryptogenic multifocal ulcerous stenosing enteritis [12], amyloidosis, Behcet's disease, pseudoxanthoma elasticum, and Ehlers-Danlos syndrome [13]. The incidence of small bowel neuroendocrine tumors (SBNET) has been increasing over the last few decades, and they are now considered as the most common primary malignancy of small bowel. Adenocarcinomas are generally seen in the proximal small bowel, whereas SBNET and lymphoma are commonly located in the distal small bowel. Sarcomas (GIST and non-GIST mesenchymal tumors: leiomyosarcoma, liposarcoma, fibrosarcoma, Kaposi's sarcoma, angiosarcoma) are evenly located throughout the small bowel.

3. Clinical presentation

Patients with mid-GI bleeding generally present with melena, occult gastrointestinal bleeding (anemia with heme-positive stool), or iron deficiency anemia. Sometimes, they may present with hematochezia as well when there is brisk mid-gut bleeding. Hematemesis is rare but can happen if bleeding occurs proximal to the ligament of Treitz. Patients can have abdominal pain, constipation, diarrhea, or constitutional symptoms like fever, anorexia, or weight loss depending on the underlying etiology. Symptoms (fatigue, shortness of breath, dysphagia due to esophageal web) and signs (pallor of conjunctiva, atrophic glossitis, and koilonychia) can be present depending on the severity and chronicity of iron deficiency anemia [14]. Patients may give history of receiving multiple blood transfusions acutely, subacutely, or chronically despite having multiple endoscopies, colonoscopies, and imaging studies.

4. Clinical evaluation

A thorough history and physical examination are essential in the evaluation of mid-GI bleeding. Besides the symptoms and signs mentioned above, there are certain clinical clues which may direct us to suspect the underlying etiology of mid-GI bleeding:

- Drug history: NSAIDs.
- Personal history: aortic stenosis (suspecting Heyde syndrome), cancer, melanoma, lymphoma, immunosuppressive state including human immunodeficiency virus (HIV) infection, celiac disease, radiation, polyposis syndrome.
- Family history: early colorectal cancer or endometrial cancer (suspecting Lynch syndrome).
- Hyperpigmentation around the mouth and on the lips, fingers, or toes may suggest Peutz-Jeghers syndrome.

- Telangiectasia on the lips and tongue may suggest hereditary hemorrhagic telangiectasia.
- Itchy blistering rash on the extensor aspect of the elbows, knees, buttocks, back, and scalp may suggest dermatitis herpetiformis.
- Cutaneous Kaposi's sarcoma.
- Oral aphthous ulcers, genital ulcers, and uveitis may suggest Behcet's syndrome.
- Cutaneous manifestations of pseudoxanthoma elasticum and Ehlers-Danlos syndrome.

5. Investigations

The various investigations used for management of mid-GI bleeding include wireless video capsule endoscopy (VCE), push enteroscopy, device-assisted enteroscopy (DAE), multiphasic CT enterography (CTE), magnetic resonance enterography (MRE), bleeding scan, Meckel's scan, angiography, and rarely laparoscopy with intraoperative enteroscopy [15–18].

5.1 VCE

VCE has revolutionized the visualization of the entire mucosa of the small bowel. It was approved by the US Food and Drug Administration (FDA) in 2001. The video capsule (size: 13 × 27.9 mm) takes 2 pictures per second with a total of approximately 57,600 color pictures wirelessly over a period of 8 hours [19]. It can detect subtle mucosal changes which cannot be detected by imaging studies. VCE is very useful not only in patients with chronic or intermittent mid-GI bleeding but also in acute overt mid-GI bleeding. VCE should be done as soon as possible after the bleeding episode ideally within 14 days in the case of chronic or recurrent overt mid-GI bleeding and within 24–72 hours of acute overt mid-GI bleeding for maximal diagnostic yield [20]. The European Society of Gastrointestinal Endoscopy (ESGE) recommends that patients should take 2 L of polyethylene glycol (PEG) and simethicone (80–200 mg) prior to VCE. Prokinetic drugs (metoclopramide or domperidone) should be given if the video capsule stays in the stomach for more than 30–60 minutes as shown by real-time VCE viewer [21, 22]. Ideally video capsule should be placed endoscopically into the small bowel by using a capsule endoscope delivery device in patients with dysphagia or abnormal gastrointestinal anatomy or delayed gastric emptying where there will be increased risk of incomplete VCE study [23]. It is safe to perform VCE in patients with cardiac pacemaker, automatic implantable cardioverter-defibrillator (AICD), and left ventricular assist device [24].

5.2 Push enteroscopy

Push enteroscopy is a very useful tool in the evaluation of lesion seen in the proximal part of the small bowel by VCE. Push enteroscopy is generally done by a dedicated push enteroscope (250 cm long) or a pediatric or standard colonoscope. Gastric looping and duodenal angulation prevent advancement of the scope. An overtube back-loaded on to the scope or a stiffening wire through the biopsy channel of the scope helps prevent loop formation of the scope allowing deeper intubation of the small bowel. The actual depth of insertion of small bowel by push enteroscopy is difficult to measure but varies (120–180 cm beyond the ligament of Treitz) among endoscopists and patients [25]. Push enteroscopy has both diagnostic and therapeutic potential including biopsy, hemostasis, and tattooing [26].

5.3 DAE

DAE includes balloon-assisted enteroscopy (single balloon and double balloon) and spiral enteroscopy.

Single-balloon enteroscopy (SBE) and double-balloon enteroscopy (DBE) were developed in 2006 and 2001, respectively, to examine the entire small bowel mucosa. Both procedures are bidirectional, i.e., the enteroscope is introduced anterogradely through the mouth and retrogradely through the anus, and the midway point is marked by tattooing or endoclipping [27]. Although the rate of complete visualization of the small bowel is three times (66 vs. 22%) higher with DBE than that with SBE [28], the diagnostic and therapeutic yields of these two procedures do not differ significantly [29]. In spiral enteroscopy (SE), the small bowel is pleated on the enteroscope by a screw operated by a machine, and the rotational force is converted into a linear force. In one study, complete enteroscopy was successful in 92% of cases of bidirectional DBE and 8% of cases of SE, although the diagnostic and therapeutic outcomes were not statistically different [30].

5.4 CTE

CTE is a useful tool in the evaluation of mid-GI bleed due to vascular lesion. Characteristic enhancement of the vascular lesion can be seen [31]. They are classified as angioectasia, arterial lesions (Dieulafoy's lesion and arteriovenous malformation), and venous lesions (vascular lesion with unusual morphology). Active bleeding is evidenced by progressive accumulation of contrast material over the three phases on the dependent surface of the intestine or distributed over a wide area by peristalsis. CT enterography is also useful in the detection of inflammatory and neoplastic condition of the small bowel [32].

5.5 MRE

MRE is a noninvasive radiation-free method of evaluating the entire small bowel. It can detect the mural thickening (>4 mm) and mass lesion of the small bowel. These lesions could be secondary to inflammatory and benign conditions (like Crohn's disease, adenoma, lipoma, fibroepithelial polyps) or malignant conditions (like neuroendocrine tumors, GIST, adenocarcinoma, lymphoma, and Peutz-Jeghers syndrome) [33, 34].

5.6 Bleeding scan

Bleeding scan is a nuclear medicine test performed by injecting 99 m technetium-labeled red blood cells (RBC). It can detect extravasation of tagged RBC if the bleeding rate is 0.1 ml/minute or more. It is a highly sensitive test in detecting active bleeding in the gastrointestinal tract and can localize the site of bleeding accurately in 52% of cases [35].

5.7 Meckel's scan

Meckel's scan is also a nuclear medicine test performed by injecting 99 m technetium pertechnetate which has affinity for the gastric mucosa. It is positive in patients with Meckel's diverticulum with heterotopic/ectopic gastric mucosa. Acid secretion from the gastric mucosa can cause ulceration and bleeding near or adjacent to the diverticulum. In children, Meckel's scan is performed early, whereas in adults, it is generally performed late in the evaluation of mid-GI bleeding.

5.8 CT angiography (CTA)

CTA is increasingly being done in patients with less brisk mid-GI bleeding. CTA can detect the bleeding site if the bleeding rate is 0.3 ml/minute or more [36]. However, CTA exposes the patient to ionizing radiation, and intravenous contrast is required. So patients with contrast allergy, renal failure, and pregnancy should avoid CTA.

5.9 Conventional mesenteric angiography (CMA)

CMA is rarely done in the evaluation of mid-GI bleeding unless there is ongoing significant bleeding and patient had hemodynamic instability, positive CTE, or bleeding scan; and embolization is considered to stop the bleeding. However, there is risk of bowel wall infarction following embolization therapy. CMA can also detect small bowel varices in patients with portal hypertension and Meckel's diverticulum by the finding of an anomalous long branch of superior mesenteric artery traversing the mesentery toward the right lower quadrant and supplying the diverticulum.

5.10 Gallium-68 dotatate PET/CT scan

Gallium-68 dotatate PET/CT scan is now considered as the best scan for detecting SBNET as 70–90% of them have somatostatin receptors. It has much better imaging quality and can detect more lesions than Octreoscan [37]. But it does not replace CTE or MRE for those SBNET which are not somatostatin receptor positive.

5.11 Intraoperative enteroscopy

Intraoperative enteroscopy is done in the operating room when other modalities of investigations fail to detect the source of bleeding. The scope is introduced through the mouth or through an enterotomy, and whole small bowel can be evaluated. It is diagnostic as well as therapeutic in achieving hemostasis in about 70% of cases.

6. Management

A systematic approach is essential to manage mid-GI successfully. Mid-GI bleeding is generally established when no source of potential bleeding is found in the upper or lower gastrointestinal tract after doing bidirectional endoscopy, i.e., upper endoscopy (including examination with a side-viewing duodenoscope) and ileocolonoscopy. Second-look bidirectional endoscopy should be done considering substantial initial endoscopic miss rates [38]. Next step to evaluate is whether the patient is hemodynamically stable or unstable and whether the patient is having occult or overt GI bleeding. The first investigation to evaluate mid-GI bleeding in a hemodynamically stable patient is VCE unless there are contraindications like small bowel obstruction [39]. On the other hand, in a hemodynamically unstable patient, the first investigation will be angiography for both diagnostic and therapeutic purposes [40].

Depending on the location of bleeding lesion in VCE, push enteroscopy or DAE should be done, i.e., push enteroscopy for lesion in the proximal part of the small bowel and DAE for lesion in the mid or distal part of the small bowel. If the VCE is negative, the next step will depend on whether the patient has ongoing blood loss, the rate of blood loss, and the presence of comorbidities:

a. If the patient has ongoing blood loss without significant comorbidities, DAE, CTE/MRE, or even laparoscopy with intraoperative enteroscopy should be considered to stop the bleeding.

b. If the patient does not have ongoing blood loss, further evaluation can be stopped.

c. If the patient has significant comorbidities and slow rate of blood loss, further investigation could be reasonably stopped. Patient should be observed with periodic monitoring of complete blood count (CBC), and iron supplementation and/or blood transfusion should be given as necessary basis.

Definitive therapy should be given according to the findings seen in the above investigations. Treatment modalities of some of the common conditions are listed below:

- Small bowel angioectasia: it is by far the commonest cause of mid-GI bleeding. Endoscopic ablation is the treatment of choice. Sometimes patients may present with recurrent anemia due to bleeding from widespread or inaccessible angioectasia, and endoscopic treatment is risky because of patients' comorbidities or old age. Pharmacologic treatment is generally offered in those cases. Thalidomide prevents angiogenesis by inhibiting vascular endothelial growth factor (VEGF). One study showed that thalidomide was effective in reducing the rate of recurrent small bowel bleeding due to vascular malformations [41]. Octreotide decreases mesenteric blood flow, inhibits angiogenesis, and improves platelet aggregation. One meta-analysis showed that octreotide therapy reduced the transfusion requirement in patients with recurrent bleeding from gastrointestinal vascular malformations [42]. Other treatment modalities for different conditions include:

- Isolated jejunal and ileal bleeding ulcers due to NSAIDs: hold NSAIDs, endoscopic treatment, and/or embolization. In rat model, proton pump inhibitors were found to worsen NSAID-induced small bowel injury by inducing dysbiosis [43].

- Dieulafoy's lesion: endoscopic (argon plasma coagulation, hemoclip, injection therapy) or angiographic intervention (embolization) or surgery if those interventions fail [44].

- Small bowel varices: endoscopic treatment if within reach of endoscope. Angiography, transjugular intrahepatic portosystemic shunt (TIPS) placement, or surgery if endoscopic hemostasis fails or is beyond the reach of endoscope [45].

- SBNET: surgical resection is the treatment of choice for locoregional disease. Long-acting somatostatin analogs are given for functional and nonfunctional metastatic SBNET because of their antiproliferative effects and ability to control carcinoid symptoms [46].

- Adenocarcinoma of small bowel: surgery, chemotherapy, and checkpoint inhibitors.
- GIST: surgery and tyrosine kinase inhibitors.
- Non-GIST mesenchymal tumors: surgery.
- Benign tumors:

  Adenoma: endoscopic resection.

  Lipoma, leiomyoma, and hamartomas: segmental resection.

  Peutz-Jeghers syndrome: segmental resection or endoscopic resection. Because some patients are young with widespread polyps, endoscopic treatment should be preferred [47].
- Metastatic tumor to the small bowel: palliative treatment.
- Meckel's diverticulum: surgery.
- Crohn's disease: endoscopic treatment, embolization, corticosteroid, 5-aminosalicylic acid, 6-mercaptopurine/azathioprine, infliximab, and surgery [48].
- Ulcerative jejunoileitis due to celiac disease: surgical resection of the ulcerated segment, corticosteroid, elimination diet, and total parenteral nutrition.

7. Prognosis

Prognosis depends on the etiology of the lesion causing mid-GI bleeding. Vascular lesions carry a good prognosis if they can be successfully treated endoscopically, radiologically, or surgically. Most of the time, vascular lesions can be managed endoscopically. Surgical intervention is required if the bleeding cannot be managed endoscopically or by interventional radiology. Surgery is also required for benign and malignant small bowel tumors, ulcerative jejunoileitis due to celiac disease, and refractory bleeding Crohn's ulcers. Sometimes, patients' comorbidities or old age do not allow invasive procedures or surgery. Symptomatic and palliative treatments are offered in those cases. Sometimes, mid-GI bleeding remains obscure. Patients end up getting multiple hospitalizations, multiple diagnostic tests, and multiple blood transfusions.

8. Conclusion

Mid-GI bleeding is common in our day-to-day clinical practice. Capsule endoscopy and imaging studies have made the diagnostic evaluations much easier than before. Balloon-assisted enteroscopy and spiral enteroscopy are generally done for therapeutic interventions. Interventional radiology and surgery are required if there is massive bleeding or endoscopic therapeutic interventions fail. After hemostasis is obtained, treatment of the underlying condition should be done. Patient's age, comorbidities, pros and cons of the procedures, and radiological and surgical interventions should be considered.

Author details

Monjur Ahmed
Thomas Jefferson University, Philadelphia, PA, USA

*Address all correspondence to: monjur.ahmed@jefferson.edu

References

[1] Ell C, May A. Mid-gastrointestinal bleeding: Capsule endoscopy and push-and-pull enteroscopy give rise to a new medical term. Endoscopy. 2006;**38**(1):73-75

[2] Murphy B, Winter DC, Kavanagh DO. Small bowel gastrointestinal bleeding diagnosis and management–A narrative review. Frontiers in Surgery. 2019;**6**:25

[3] Gunjan D, Sharma V, Rana SS, Bhasin DK. Small bowel bleeding: A comprehensive review. Gastroenterology Report. 2014;**2**(4):262-275

[4] Gerson LB, Fidler JL, Cave DR, Leighton JA. ACG clinical guideline: Diagnosis and management of small bowel bleeding. The American Journal of Gastroenterology. 2015;**110**(9):1265-1287

[5] Song JH, Hong SN, Kyung Chang D, Ran Jeon S, Kim JO, Kim J, et al. The etiology of potential small-bowel bleeding depending on patient's age and gender. United European Gastroenterology Journal. 2018;**6**(8):1169-1178

[6] Katz LB. The role of surgery in occult gastrointestinal bleeding. Seminars in Gastrointestinal Disease. 1999;**10**(2):78-81

[7] Raju GS, Gerson L, Das A, Lewis B, American Gastroenterological Association. American Gastroenterological Association (AGA) institute medical position statement on obscure gastrointestinal bleeding. Gastroenterology. 2007;**133**(5):1694-1696

[8] Shi X, Yu S, Wang F, Zhao Q, Xu H, Li B. A gastrointestinal stromal tumor with acute bleeding: Management and nursing. Medicine. 2018;**97**(9):e9874

[9] Yatagai N, Ueyama H, Shibuya T, Haga K, Takahashi M, Nomura O, et al. Obscure gastrointestinal bleeding caused by small intestinal lipoma: A case report. Journal of Medical Case Reports. 2016;**10**(1):226

[10] Zheng W, Song Y, Lin N, Tu M, Liu W, Zhu J. Primary gastrointestinal mantle lymphoma with massive bleeding: A case report and literature review. Chinese Journal of Cancer Research. 2013;**25**(2):250-253

[11] Kreis DJ Jr, Guerra JJ Jr, Saltz M, Santiesteban R, Byers P. Gastrointestinal hemorrhage due to carcinoid tumors of the small intestine. Journal of the American Medical Association. 1986;**255**(2):234-236

[12] Hwang J, Kim JS, Kim AY, Lim JS, Kim SH, Kim MJ, et al. Cryptogenic multifocal ulcerous stenosing enteritis: Radiologic features and clinical behavior. World Journal of Gastroenterology. 2017;**23**(25):4615-4623

[13] Allaparthi S, Verma H, Burns DL, Joyce AM. Conservative management of small bowel perforation in Ehlers-Danlos syndrome type IV. World Journal of Gastrointestinal Endoscopy. 2013;**5**(8):398-401

[14] Samad A, Mohan N, Balaji RV, Augustine D, Patil SG. Oral manifestations of Plummer-Vinson syndrome: A classic report with literature review. Journal of International Oral Health. 2015;**7**(3):68-71

[15] ASGE Standards of Practice Committee, Gurudu SR, Bruining DH, Acosta RD, Eloubeidi MA, Faulx AL, et al. The role of endoscopy in the management of suspected small-bowel bleeding. Gastrointestinal Endoscopy. 2017;**85**(1):22-31

[16] Lee SS, Oh TS, Kim HJ, Chung JW, Park SH, Kim AY, et al. Obscure gastrointestinal bleeding: Diagnostic performance of multidetector CT enterography. Radiology. 2011;**259**(3):739-748

[17] Masselli G, Gualdi G. MR imaging of the small bowel. Radiology. 2012;**264**(2):333-348

[18] Lewis BS, Wenger JS, Waye JD. Small bowel enteroscopy and intraoperative enteroscopy for obscure gastrointestinal bleeding. The American Journal of Gastroenterology. 1991;**86**(2):171-174

[19] Raju GS, Gerson L, Das A, Lewis B, American Gastroenterological Association. American Gastroenterological Association (AGA) institute technical review on obscure gastrointestinal bleeding. Gastroenterology. 2007;**133**(5):1697-1717

[20] Pennazio M, Spada C, Eliakim R, Keuchel M, May A, Mulder CJ, et al. Small-bowel capsule endoscopy and device-assisted enteroscopy for diagnosis and treatment of small-bowel disorders: European Society of Gastrointestinal Endoscopy (ESGE) clinical guideline. Endoscopy. 2015;**47**(4):352-376

[21] Koulaouzidis A, Giannakou A, Yung DE, Dabos KJ, Plevris JN. Do prokinetics influence the completion rate in small-bowel capsule endoscopy? A systematic review and meta-analysis. Current Medical Research and Opinion. 2013;**29**(9):1171-1185

[22] Lai LH, Wong GL, Lau JY, Sung JJ, Leung WK. Initial experience of real-time capsule endoscopy in monitoring progress of the videocapsule through the upper GI tract. Gastrointestinal Endoscopy. 2007;**66**(6):1211-1214

[23] Holden JP, Dureja P, Pfau PR, Schwartz DC, Reichelderfer M, Judd RH, et al. Endoscopic placement of the small-bowel video capsule by using a capsule endoscope delivery device. Gastrointestinal Endoscopy. 2007;**65**(6):842-847

[24] Rondonotti E, Spada C, Adler S, May A, Despott EJ, Koulaouzidis A, et al. Small-bowel capsule endoscopy and device-assisted enteroscopy for diagnosis and treatment of small-bowel disorders: European Society of Gastrointestinal Endoscopy (ESGE) technical review. Endoscopy. 2018;**50**(4):423-446

[25] Barth B. Capsule endoscopy and small bowel enteroscopy. In: Wyllie R, Hyams JS, editors. Pediatric Gastrointestinal and Liver Disease. 4th ed. Philadelphia: Elsevier; 2011. pp. 679-685.e2. ISBN: 978-1-4377-0774-8. https://doi.org/10.1016/C2009-0-53242-4

[26] Kovacs TO. Small bowel bleeding. Current Treatment Options in Gastroenterology. 2005;**8**(1):31-38

[27] Kawamura T, Uno K, Tanaka K, Yasuda K. Current status of single-balloon enteroscopy: Insertability and clinical applications. World Journal of Gastrointestinal Endoscopy. 2015;**7**(1):59-65

[28] May A, Färber M, Aschmoneit I, Pohl J, Manner H, Lotterer E, et al. Prospective multicenter trial comparing push-and-pull enteroscopy with the single- and double-balloon techniques in patients with small-bowel disorders. The American Journal of Gastroenterology. 2010;**105**(3):575-581

[29] Prachayakul V, Deesomsak M, Aswakul P, Leelakusolvong S. The utility of single-balloon enteroscopy for the diagnosis and management of small bowel disorders according to their clinical manifestations: A retrospective review. BMC Gastroenterology. 2013;**13**:103

[30] Akerman PA. Spiral enteroscopy versus double-balloon enteroscopy: Choosing the right tool for the job. Gastrointestinal Endoscopy. 2013;**77**(2):252-254

[31] Huprich JE, Barlow JM, Hansel SL, Alexander JA, Fidler JL. Multiphase CT enterography evaluation of small-bowel vascular lesions. AJR. American Journal of Roentgenology. 2013;**201**(1):65-72

[32] Masselli G. Small bowel imaging: Clinical applications of the different imaging modalities—A comprehensive review. ISRN Pathology. 2013;**2013**:419542, 13 p. DOI: 10.1155/2013/419542

[33] Cengic I, Tureli D, Aydin H, Bugdayci O, Imeryuz N, Tuney D. Magnetic resonance enterography in refractory iron deficiency anemia: A pictorial overview. World Journal of Gastroenterology. 2014;**20**(38):14004-14009

[34] Kumar AS, Coralic J, Vegeler R, Kolli K, Liang J, Estep A, et al. Magnetic resonance enterography: The test of choice in diagnosing intestinal "zebras". Case Reports in Gastrointestinal Medicine. 2015;**2015**:206469

[35] Bentley DE, Richardson JD. The role of tagged red blood cell imaging in the localization of gastrointestinal bleeding. Archives of Surgery. 1991;**126**(7):821-824

[36] García-Blázquez V, Vicente-Bártulos A, Olavarria-Delgado A, Plana MN, van der Winden D, Zamora J, et al. Accuracy of CT angiography in the diagnosis of acute gastrointestinal bleeding: Systematic review and meta-analysis. European Radiology. 2013;**23**(5):1181-1190

[37] Mojtahedi A, Thamake S, Tworowska I, Ranganathan D, Delpassand ES. The value of (68) Ga-DOTATATE PET/CT in diagnosis and management of neuroendocrine tumors compared to current FDA approved imaging modalities: A review of literature. American Journal of Nuclear Medicine and Molecular Imaging. 2014;**4**(5):426-434. eCollection 2014

[38] Fry LC, Bellutti M, Neumann H, Malfertheiner P, Mönkemüller K. Incidence of bleeding lesions within reach of conventional upper and lower endoscopes in patients undergoing double-balloon enteroscopy for obscure gastrointestinal bleeding. Alimentary Pharmacology & Therapeutics. 2009;**29**(3):342-349

[39] Leung WK, Ho SS, Suen BY, Lai LH, Yu S, Ng EK, et al. Capsule endoscopy or angiography in patients with acute overt obscure gastrointestinal bleeding: A prospective randomized study with long-term follow-up. The American Journal of Gastroenterology. 2012;**107**(9):1370

[40] Walker TG, Salazar GM, Waltman AC. Angiographic evaluation and management of acute gastrointestinal hemorrhage. World Journal of Gastroenterology. 2012;**18**(11):1191-1201

[41] Ge ZZ, Chen HM, Gao YJ, Liu WZ, Xu CH, Tan HH, et al. Efficacy of thalidomide for refractory gastrointestinal bleeding from vascular malformation. Gastroenterology. 2011;**141**(5):1629-37.e1-4

[42] Brown C, Subramanian V, Wilcox CM, Peter S. Somatostatin analogues in the treatment of recurrent bleeding from gastrointestinal vascular malformations: An overview and systematic review of prospective observational studies. Digestive Diseases and Sciences. 2010;**55**(8):2129-2134

[43] Wallace JL, Syer S, Denou E, de Palma G, Vong L, McKnight W, et al.

Proton pump inhibitors exacerbate NSAID-induced small intestinal injury by inducing dysbiosis. Gastroenterology. 2011;**141**(4):1314-1322, 1322.e1-5

[44] Baxter M, Aly EH. Dieulafoy's lesion: Current trends in diagnosis and management. Annals of the Royal College of Surgeons of England. 2010;**92**(7):548-554

[45] Norton ID, Andrews JC, Kamath PS. Management of ectopic varices. Hepatology. 1998;**28**(4):1154-1158

[46] Scott AT, Howe JR. Management of small bowel neuroendocrine tumors. Journal of Oncology Practice. 2018;**14**(8):471-482

[47] Wang R, Qi X, Shao X, Guo X. A large intracolonic mass in a patient with Peutz-Jeghers syndrome. Middle East Journal of Digestive Diseases. 2017;**9**(3):173-175

[48] Podugu A, Tandon K, Castro FJ. Crohn's disease presenting as acute gastrointestinal hemorrhage. World Journal of Gastroenterology. 2016;**22**(16):4073-4078

Chapter 3

Gastrointestinal Manifestations of IgA Vasculitis-Henoch-Schönlein Purpura

Camelia Cojocariu, Ana Maria Singeap, Stefan Chiriac, Catalin Sfarti, Irina Girleanu, Oana Petrea, Anca Trifan and Carol Stanciu

Abstract

Immunoglobulin A vasculitis, formerly called Henoch-Schönlein purpura (HSP), is the most common systemic vasculitis in childhood. It is a small-vessel vasculitis mediated by type III hypersensitivity, manifested as rash accompanied by gastrointestinal (GI) symptoms, arthritis, and nephritis. The etiology of this disease (a leukocytoclastic vasculitis) is still uncertain, but immune complexes of IgA and unidentified antigens seem to have a central pathogenic role. Most often the diagnosis is established after the clinical examination; it is easy at first glance when the clinical presentation includes the classic tetrad of rash (nonthrombocytopenic palpable purpura), arthralgia/arthritis, abdominal pain, and renal manifestations but may be difficult when the gastrointestinal manifestations precede the skin purpuric rash. Gastrointestinal involvement is frequently seen and varies from mild symptoms to severe complications; sometimes the gastrointestinal symptoms (colicky abdominal pain, nausea, vomiting, diarrhea, gastrointestinal bleeding) are the first manifestations of the disease. Immunoglobulin A vasculitis is usually a self-limited disease with a benign course, and the treatment is often symptomatic; in severe cases corticosteroids are necessary.

Keywords: Henoch-Schönlein purpura, IgA vasculitis, gastrointestinal involvement

1. Introduction

In 1837 Schönlein described a clinical triad manifested as purpuric rash, arthralgias/arthritis, and renal involvement; 1 year later, Henoch related the association of rash, abdominal pain (with bloody diarrhea), and proteinuria; the clinical association of these symptoms was diagnosed as Henoch-Schönlein purpura.

The term Henoch-Schönlein purpura was replaced with immunoglobulin A vasculitis (IgA vasculitis), by the 2012 revised Chapel Hill International Consensus Conference for Nomenclature of Vasculitides [1], based on IgA1-dominant immune deposits affecting small vessels and typically involving the skin, joints, gastrointestinal tract, and kidney.

Henoch-Schönlein purpura (HSP) is a small-vessel vasculitis, characterized by a generalized vascular involvement, usually involving the small vessels of the skin, the gastrointestinal (GI) tract, the kidneys, and the joints; it is an acute IgA-mediated disorder that rarely may affect the lungs and the central nervous system (CNS) [2]. IgA vasculitis is a multi-system disorder characterized by palpable purpura, arthritis, glomerulonephritis, and gastrointestinal manifestations and is the most common form of systemic vasculitis for children (90% of cases occur in the pediatric patients) [3].

Although a lot of algorithm diagnoses were proposed (The American College of Rheumatology, Michel's criteria, Chapel Hill Consensus Conference, etc.) [1], the diagnostic criteria remain the one published in 2006 [4], revised by the European League Against Rheumatism/Pediatric Rheumatology International Trial Organization/Pediatric Rheumatology European Society (EULAR/PRINTO/PRES); the mandatory criterion is palpable purpura in association with at least one of the following: diffuse abdominal pain, arthritis or arthralgia, renal involvement (hematuria and/or proteinuria), and IgA deposition in biopsy specimen (skin, intestinal tract) [5].

Differential diagnosis includes many diseases with systemic manifestations (cutaneous, articular, gastrointestinal, renal) such as Crohn's disease (no palpable purpura or gastrointestinal bleeding), IgA nephropathy (no palpable purpura), and hypersensitivity vasculitis (absence of IgA deposition) [4].

2. Epidemiology

IgA vasculitis is the most common vasculitis for children; it is usually seen in children between 3 and 10 years old (the age peak is 5–7 years) and very rarely in adults [3, 4]. The annual incidence varies greatly, from 13 to 20/100,000 for children to 0.8–1.8/100,000 for adults [6–8]. Demographic data showed that males are more frequently affected (male-to-female ratio varies from 1.2:1 to 1.8:1) [3, 9].

The diagnosis is more commonly established in winter and spring and rarely in summer [7, 8], and this aspect may be explained by the association of this disease with infection factors, while approximately 50% of IgA cases are preceded by an upper respiratory tract infection [10].

Clinical features and severity of the disease also differ by aging, being more severe in adults than in children [10].

3. Pathogenesis

IgA vasculitis is a small-vessel vasculitis syndrome involving the small vessels of the skin, gastrointestinal tract, kidneys, and joints, consisting of palpable purpura, arthralgia, and gastrointestinal and renal manifestations.

The etiology is still unknown, but precipitating factors such as drug intake and/or upper respiratory tract infections have been associated with the disease development [11]. Although a variety of infectious and chemical triggers are recognized, the underlying cause remains unknown.

In approximately two-thirds of the cases, typical symptoms occur after 7–14 days from an upper respiratory tract infection (previous epidemiological studies have found a seasonal variation of incidence in IgA vasculitis, with more cases occurring in autumn and winter related with upper respiratory tract infection) [4, 11].

Other cases of IgA vasculitis have been associated with several viral infections or vaccinations, foods, drugs, hematological malignancies, and tumors [4].

Henoch-Schönlein purpura (HSP) is mediated by type III hypersensitivity with deposition of IgA immune complex in the walls of vessels.

Histologically, this disease is characterized by leukocytoclastic vasculitis accompanied by IgA immune complexes within affected organs (deposition of IgA and C3 in small-vessel walls, polymorphonuclear leukocyte infiltration around/in small blood vessels, and leukocytoclasia) [11]. The biopsy of the purpuric lesions showed the involvement of small vessels (primarily postcapillary venules) within the papillary dermis and that the predominant cell types within the inflammatory infiltrate are neutrophils and monocytes [12].

Although the pathogenesis of the disease remains unknown, several authors confirmed the implication of abnormal glycosylation of the hinge region of IgA1, elevated levels of IgA anticardiolipin antibodies, and increased levels of transforming growth factor (TGF)-beta in patients with Ig A vasculitis [12, 13].

The diagnosis is often a clinical one (based on the classic symptoms and signs); since there is no disease-specific laboratory abnormality, no specific test available was able to establish the diagnosis.

4. Clinical manifestation

IgA vasculitis typically has a prodrome (headache, anorexia, fever); after that, a lot of symptoms may develop: rash (especially involving the legs), abdominal pain and vomiting, joint pain (especially involving the knees and ankles), subcutaneous edema, scrotal edema, etc.

The classic tetrad symptoms are rash, arthralgia/arthritis, abdominal pain, and renal manifestations. The clinical diagnosis is easily made in the presence of all these symptoms but may be omitted when the clinical picture is incomplete; in the absence of the classic purpuric rash, the diagnosis of Ig A vasculitis may not be obvious [14, 15].

Purpura and joint pain are usually the main symptoms on admission, but the symptoms may develop over the course of some days to weeks and may vary in their order of presentation.

The major clinical manifestations are the following:

- Purpura—the appearing symptom in approximately 75% of patients, usually preceding other symptoms
- Arthralgia/arthritis—50–75% of cases
- Abdominal pain—colicky pain in 50% of cases and gastrointestinal bleeding in 20–30% of cases
- Renal disease—20–50% [6, 11, 16–18]

4.1 Skin manifestation

The skin lesions are the earliest and most common appearance of the disease in the majority of patients (70%) and include palpable nonthrombocytopenic purpura which evolves from erythema to papules and then to non-blanching palpable purpura with petechiae and ecchymosis (**Figure 1**). The rash is the hallmark of the disease and typically appears in crops, with new crops appearing in waves (eruptions usually last an average of 3 weeks).

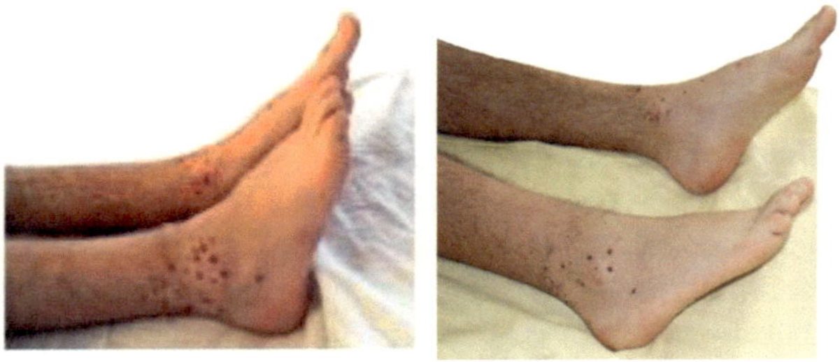

Figure 1.
Palpable purpura on both ankles.

The typical rash is symmetrically distributed and located primarily in gravity-/pressure-dependent areas, such as the feet, ankles, and lower legs in adults; in the case of children, the buttocks, face, trunk, and upper extremities are more affected [19]. In child patients purpura gradually disappears (it can recur and become chronic), but in adults, it may be necrotic or hemorrhagic in 1/3 of cases, and cutaneous exacerbations may be seen for 6 months or longer [20, 21].

4.2 Joint involvement

Arthralgia or arthritis is present in 2/3 of cases of patients; joint complaints are uncommon as the first symptom, but it is the appearing complaint in approximately 25% of children [21]. The articular manifestations are seen more often in adults than in children; typically involve the hips, knees, and ankles (less commonly the upper extremities); and are symmetrical (as skin lesions) in distribution [4]. The joint involvement is usually transient or migratory, typically oligoarticular and non-deforming. A prominent periarticular swelling and tenderness are usual, without joint effusion, erythema, or warmth. The most frequent symptom is arthralgia, while arthritis is very rare; joint effusions are exceptional [20].

4.3 Renal involvement

Renal involvement is found in 40–85% of patients (more prevalent in older children and adults), ranging from microscopic hematuria to progressive glomerulonephritis, and is the most serious complication of Ig A vasculitis [17, 20]. The most common presentation is hematuria (with/without red blood casts) and mild proteinuria; proteinuria without hematuria is very rare. Renal manifestations usually develop within 4 weeks and never precede the onset of skin lesions. The risk of renal failure is rare in children [22] but may be present in about 30% of adult cases, especially in patients with nephrotic and nephritic syndromes [4]. Nephrotic-range proteinuria, elevated serum creatinine, hypertension, and the coexistence of hematuria and proteinuria are associated with an increased risk of renal failure; 2–5% of patients with renal involvement come to an end-stage renal failure [12, 17].

4.4 Gastrointestinal manifestations

Gastrointestinal involvement occurs in 50–75% of adult patients—abdominal pain and bloody diarrhea may precede the typical purpuric rash [15, 23]. The digestive symptoms are often present in patients with IgA vasculitis, and although less commonly found in adults, they are more severe and often atypical. The gastrointestinal symptoms vary in intensity, and prudent laparotomy is required to exclude an acute abdominal condition. Gastrointestinal manifestations range from mild (nausea, vomiting, abdominal pain, paralytic ileus) to severe findings (gastrointestinal bleeding, intussusception, bowel ischemia with secondary necrosis, bowel perforation).

Gastrointestinal symptoms are often the most debilitating manifestations of the disease, and they are much more common in younger patients than in elders [23, 24].

The gastrointestinal manifestations may precede the onset of IgA vasculitis or may develop later in the course of the disease. Typically, gastrointestinal symptoms develop within 8 days from the rash appearance, although longer periods (weeks, even months) have been described. In 10–15% of cases, the gastrointestinal symptoms occur before cutaneous manifestation, making the differential diagnosis of other causes of acute abdomen more difficult [24]. Rarely, gastrointestinal symptoms may appear with no cutaneous purpura at any time [25, 26].

Abdominal pain is the most common gastrointestinal symptom, manifested by colicky pain worsened by food (similar to bowel angina), localized to the epigastric and periumbilical regions. The pain is attributed to the involvement of the splanchnic circulation (mesenteric vasculitis) with bowel ischemia and edema of the gastrointestinal tract [4, 23, 27]. Abdominal pain associated with IgAV is caused by submucosal hemorrhage and edema.

Abdominal pain is often associated with diarrhea with gross or occult blood, nausea, vomiting, constipation, and gastrointestinal bleeding (hematemesis or melena).

In most cases, on clinical examination, the abdomen is tender and slightly distended; rarely, it may resemble and be confused with an acute abdomen requiring surgery evaluation (suspicion of perforation, intussusception). Some of these cases, suggesting an acute abdomen, are leading to emergency computed tomography (CT) or unnecessary surgery [4, 23]. Sometimes, particularly in young patients, intense abdominal pain may suggest acute appendicitis, especially when the skin rash is absent. Even in the presence of rash (suggestive in a clinical context for Ig A vasculitis) in front of intense abdominal pain, the differential diagnosis of abdominal pain and the exclusion of acute surgical abdomen are mandatory; more, the IgA vasculitis rash may be a nonspecific erythematous or urticarial exanthem or limited to lesions on the buttocks or lower extremities early in the disease course.

Gastrointestinal bleeding is another symptom, with an incidence varying between 17.6 and 51% [23]. In most cases, the bleeding is occult (detected as positive stool occult blood); when manifested, the main symptom is melena rather than hematemesis or hematochezia, because the intestinal lesions are usually localized in the small bowel and colon. Gastrointestinal bleeding is usually mild; in rare cases it may be severe, requiring blood transfusion or surgical treatment, even leading to death [4, 23].

Other rare gastrointestinal manifestations, such as *esophageal ulcer*, *pancreatitis*, *pseudomembranous colitis*, *gall bladder involvement*, *intestinal perforation*, and *ischemic vasculitis* may occur [23].

Intussusception is the most common gastrointestinal complication of IgA vasculitis. Edema and hemorrhage can act as a pathological lead point, contributing to the development of intussusception. Intussusception is limited to the small bowel in approximately 60% of cases, in contrast to idiopathic intussusception, which is typically ileocolic. The overall incidence of this complication of IgA vasculitis varies between 2.3 and 3.5%, although some retrospective series reported an incidence of only 0.4 to 0.6% [9, 17]. Children with severe gastrointestinal pain and/or requiring hospitalization are at greater risk.

4.4.1 Imaging evaluation of gastrointestinal manifestation

Upper gastrointestinal endoscopy (UGD) is mandatory in patients with gastrointestinal bleeding. UGD is helpful in the diagnosis of IgA vasculitis, especially when gastrointestinal symptoms develop prior to the cutaneous lesions.

The most important part of upper gastrointestinal tract is involved in the second part of the duodenum with endoscopic features including diffuse mucosal redness, petechiae, severe erosive duodenitis, hemorrhagic lesion, and ulcers [28] (**Figure 2**). Purpuric lesions may be seen on an endoscopy, commonly in the descending duodenum, stomach, and colon.

The spectrum of upper endoscopic findings is based upon the severity of the vasculitis; usually, irregular, ulcerating, nodular lesions or hematoma-like protrusions are characteristic of IgA vasculitis in the duodenum. The stomach and colon are often involved as well, but the duodenal bulb is rarely affected; the absence of bulbar lesions is important to exclude the cause of the peptic disease hemorrhage [29]. The biopsies of gastrointestinal lesions are commonly performed in patients with or without suspected IgA vasculitis in order to rule out infection, inflammatory bowel disease, and less commonly, vasculitis. In general, vasculitis is not commonly observed in GI biopsies, and the spectrum of findings includes neutrophilic infiltrate within the small bowel and colon, with the duodenum most commonly affected. While the clinical and histologic findings may mimic early inflammatory bowel disease, the presence of predominant small bowel involvement, especially erosive duodenitis, should raise suspicion for IgA vasculitis. Biopsies should be obtained before steroid therapy is initiated, if possible [30].

Resolution of duodenal lesions is spectacular, in accordance with the remission of inflammatory disorders [31] (**Figure 3**).

Colonoscopy: erythema of the mucosa, petechiae, and ulcers are the most common findings [32].

Computed tomography (CT) imaging: the hallmarks of IgA vasculitis are multifocal symmetric, circumferential, regular wall thickening and engorgement of mesenteric vessels. Associated findings include free intraperitoneal fluid, ileus of the affected loop, vascular engorgement in the adjoining mesentery, and nonspecific lymphadenopathy [24]. The target sign is not specific; it can be seen in many other conditions such as ischemic bowel disease, inflammatory bowel disease, infectious enterocolitis, radiation enteritis, etc. [19].

In some selected cases, CT angiography can be used to visualize the site of the arterial or venous occlusion; however, a normal angiogram does not rule out the possibility of mesenteric ischemia [3]. Mesenteric vascular engorgement and skip areas are also seen in Crohn's disease, but terminal ileal involvement, stricture, fistula, and abscess would favor Crohn's disease over other conditions [12, 33].

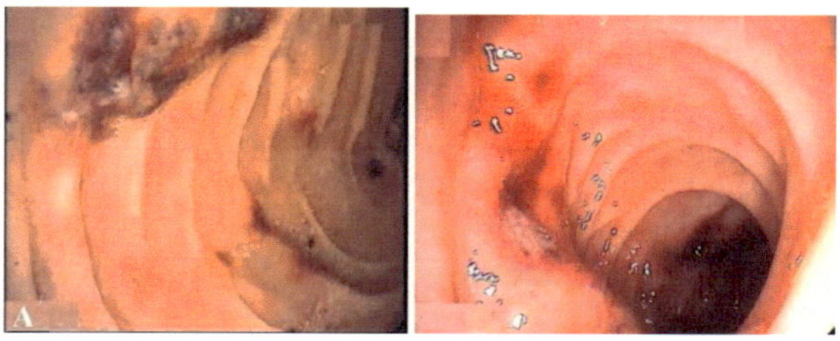

Figure 2.
Endoscopic appearance of the second part of duodenum: multiple erosions, diffuse redness, submucosal hemorrhage, and small ulcerations.

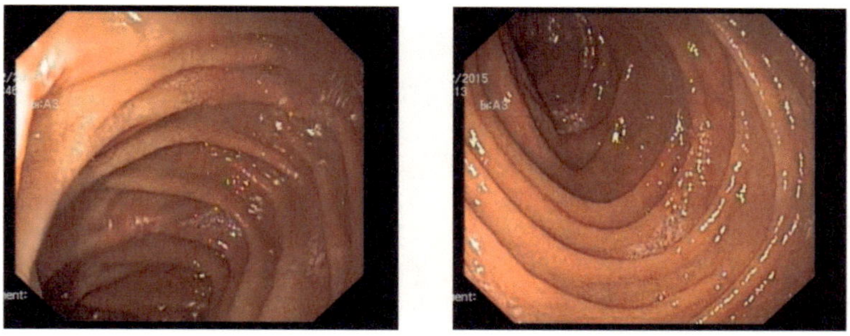

Figure 3.
Endoscopic appearance of the second part of duodenum remission.

5. Conclusion

The diagnosis of IgA vasculitis (HSP) is usually based upon clinical manifestations of the disease, and in patients with an incomplete/unusual presentation, biopsy of the affected organ (e.g., skin or kidney) demonstrating predominantly IgA deposition supports the diagnosis. Although gastrointestinal involvement is frequent, the diagnosis of IgA vasculitis may be difficult when gastrointestinal manifestations occur alone or precede the characteristic skin purpura.

Author details

Camelia Cojocariu[1,2]*, Ana Maria Singeap[1,2], Stefan Chiriac[1,2], Catalin Sfarti[1,2], Irina Girleanu[1,2], Oana Petrea[1,2], Anca Trifan[1,2] and Carol Stanciu[2]

1 University of Medicine and Pharmacy "Gr. T. Popa", Iasi, Romania

2 "St. Spiridon" Emergency Hospital, Institute of Gastroenterology and Hepatology, Iasi, Romania

*Address all correspondence to: cameliacojocariu@yahoo.com

References

[1] Jennette JC, Falk RJ, Bacon PA, et al. 2012 Revised International Chapel Hill Consensus Conference Nomenclature of Vasculitides. Arthritis and Rheumatism. 2013;**65**(1):1-11

[2] Szer IS. Henoch-Schönlein purpura. Current Opinion in Rheumatology. 1994;**6**(1):25-31

[3] Piram M, Mahr A. Epidemiology of immunoglobulin A vasculitis (Henoch-Schönlein): Current state of knowledge. Current Opinion in Rheumatology. 2013;**25**:171

[4] Ebert EC. Gastrointestinal manifestation of Henoch Schönlein purpura. Digestive Diseases and Sciences. 2008;**53**:2011-2019

[5] Yang YH, Yu HH, Chiang BL. The diagnosis and classification of Henoch-Schönlein purpura: An updated review. Autoimmunity Reviews. 2014;**13**(4-5):355-358

[6] Gardner-Medwin J, Dolezalova P, Cummins C, Southwood TR. Incidence of Henoch-Schönlein purpura, Kawasaki disease, and rare vasculitides in children of different ethnic origins. Lancet. 2002;**360**(9):1197-1202

[7] Watts RA, Lane S, Scott DG. What is known about the epidemiology of the vasculitides? Best Practice & Research. Clinical Rheumatology. 2005;**19**:191-207

[8] Blanco R, Martínez-Taboada VM, Rodríguez-Valverde V, et al. Henoch-Schönlein purpura in adulthood and childhood: Two different expressions of the same syndrome. Arthritis and Rheumatism. 1997;**40**:859

[9] Trapani S, Micheli A, Grisolia F, et al. Henoch Schonlein purpura in childhood: Epidemiological and clinical analysis of 150 cases over a 5-year period and review of literature. Seminars in Arthritis and Rheumatism. 2005;**35**:143

[10] Schaier M, Freitag J, Dikow R, et al. Henoch-Schönlein purpura in adults is not uncommon in elderly patients with an adverse prognosis. Clinical Nephrology. 2011;**76**:49-56

[11] Calvo Rio V, Loricera J, Mata C, et al. Henoch-Schönlein purpura in northern Spain: Clinical spectrum of the disease in 417 patients from a single center. Medicine (Baltimore). 2014;**93**(2):106-113

[12] Dedeoglu F, Kim S. IgA Vasculitis (Henoch-Schönlein purpura): Clinical Manifestations and Diagnosis. Available from: https://www.uptodate.com/contents/iga-vasculitis-henoch-schonlein-purpura-clinical-manifestations-and-diagnosis

[13] Lau KK, Wyatt RJ, Moldoveanu Z, et al. Serum levels of galactose-deficient IgA in children with IgA nephropathy and Henoch-Schönlein purpura. Pediatric Nephrology. 2007;**22**:2067

[14] Saulsbury FT. Clinical update: Henoch-Schönlein purpura. Lancet. 2007;**369**:976-978

[15] Cojocariu C, Stanciu C, Ancuta C, Danciu M, Chiriac S, Trifan A. Immunoglobulin A vasculitis complicated with clostridium difficile infection: A rare case report and brief review of the literature. Journal of Gastrointestinal and Liver Diseases. 2016;**25**(2):235-238

[16] Kang Y, Park JS, Ha YJ, et al. Differences in clinical manifestations and outcomes between adult and child patients with Henoch-Schönlein purpura. Journal of Korean Medical Science. 2014;**29**:198

[17] Ghrahani R, Ledika MA, Sapartini G, Setiabudiawan B. Age of onset as

a risk factor of renal involvement in Henoch-Schönlein purpura. Asia Pacific Allergy. 2014;**4**:42

[18] Peru H, Soylemezoglu O, Bakkaloglu SA, et al. Henoch Schonlein purpura in childhood: Clinical analysis of 254 cases over a 3-year period. Clinical Rheumatology. 2008;**27**:1087

[19] Audemand-Verger A, Pillebout E, Guillevin L, Thervet E, Terrier B. IgA vasculitis (Henoch-Schönlein purpura) in adults: Diagnostic and therapeutic aspects. Autoimmunity Reviews. 2015;**14**:579-585

[20] Pilebout E. Adult Henoch-Schönlein purpura. Presse Médicale. 2008;**37**(12):1773-1778

[21] Thrash B, Patel M, Shah KR, Boland CR, Menter A. Cutaneous manifestations of gastrointestinal disease: Part II. Journal of the American Academy of Dermatology. 2013;**68**(2):211.e1-211.e33

[22] Selewski DT, Ambruzs JM, Appel GB, et al. Clinical characteristics and treatment patterns of children and adults with IgA nephropathy or IgA vasculitis: Findings from the CureGN Study. Kidney International Reports. 2018;**3**(6):1373-1384

[23] Hamzaoui A, Melki W, Harzallah O, et al. Gastrointestinal involvement revealing Henoch Schonlein purpura in adults: Report of three cases and review of the literature. International Archives of Medicine. 2011;**4**:31

[24] Rajalakshmi PP, Srinivasan K. Gastrointestinal manifestations of Henoch-Schönlein purpura: A report of two cases. World Journal of Radiology. 2015;7(3):66-69

[25] Nathan K, Gunasekaran TS, Berman JH. Recurrent gastrointestinal Henoch-Schönlein purpura. Journal of Clinical Gastroenterology. 1999;**29**:86

[26] Gunasekaran TS, Berman J, Gonzalez M. Duodenojejunitis: Is it idiopathic or is it Henoch-Schönlein purpura without the purpura? Journal of Pediatric Gastroenterology and Nutrition. 2000;**30**:22

[27] Sohagia BA, Gunturu GS, Tong RT, Hertan LH. Henoch-Schönlein purpura—A case report and review of literature. Gastroenterology Research and Practice. 2010;**2010**:7

[28] Chen XL, Tian H, Li JZ, et al. Paroxysmal drastic abdominal pain with tardive cutaneous lesions presenting in Henoch-Schönlein purpura. World Journal of Gastroenterology. 2012;**18**(16):1991-1995

[29] Dharmesh K, Chodos A, Ahlawat S. Henoch-Schonlein purpura with gastrointestinal involvement in an adult patient. Gastroenterología y Hepatología. 2016;**12**(5):321-323

[30] Louie CY, Gomez AJ, et al. Histologic features of gastrointestinal tract biopsies in IgA vasculitis (Henoch-Schönlein Purpura). The American Journal of Surgical Pathology. 2018;**42**(4):529-533

[31] Rubino C, Paci M, Resti M, Lionetti P, Trapani S. Late relapse of Henoch-Schönlein purpura in an adolescent presenting as severe gastroduodenitis. Frontiers in Pediatrics. 2018;**6**:355

[32] Huang L, Sun L, Lu C, et al. Endoscopy and the management of IgA vasculitis: A clinical analysis of 261 pediatric immunoglobulin A (IgA) vasculitis cases with gastrointestinal involvement and endoscopic examinations of 69 patients. International Journal of Clinical and Experimental Medicine. 2019;**12**(2):2035-2041

[33] Hočevar A, Rotar Z, Ostrovršnik J, et al. Incidence of IgA vasculitis in the adult Slovenian population. The British Journal of Dermatology. 2014;**171**:524

Chapter 4

Biomechanics of the Small Intestinal Contractions

Ravi Kant Avvari

Abstract

The small intestine is a part of the gastrointestinal segment comprising of the duodenum, jejunum, and ileum. They help to process the gastric contents for further digestion, which involves mixing with duodeno-biliary-pancreatic (DBP) secretions to facilitate the chemical digestion, and homogenization of the luminal contents through contractions of the circular and longitudinal smooth muscle fibers of the intestine. The contractions of these smooth muscle fibers develops the mechanical forces at the mucosal wall, which as a consequence, transfers its momentum to the underlying fluid to develop the fluid flows, suggesting relevance of mechanics in physiology. The resulting flows are what drive the digestion. Changes in contractility of wave shapes of circular and longitudinal smooth muscle contractions and fluid rheology are known to affect the digestive process through generation of various flow patterns that differ in luminal pressure, peak velocity, extent of shearing/ mixing, volume of mixing, and flow rate. Recent studies indicate that the digestive process can be very specific such as to cause lipid digestion through segmental contractions and transport by eliciting propagating contractions, suggesting that the intestine manages to digest a variety of food in an efficient manner by eliciting appropriate contractions.

Keywords: small intestine, small intestinal motility, peristalsis, circular contraction, local longitudinal shortening

1. Introduction

The human small intestine is a part of the gastrointestinal tract which extends from end of the stomach to the inlet of large intestine. They form the visceral organ of our body which helps in processing the food at various levels such as mixing, digestion (mechanical grinding and chemical breakdown), and transport. They are arranged in a complex 3D manner, having numerous folds (convolutions) and flexures. The small intestine is functionally divided into duodenum, jejunum, and ileum; each of which has a specific physiology function to play in the digestion. They enable the digestion of meal in these compartments through coordinative effort. The small intestine elicits a complex series of motility patterns depending on the nature of meal to help (1) mixing with duodeno-biliary-pancreatic (DBP) secretions to facilitate the chemical digestion, (2) homogenization of the luminal contents of intestine, (3) regulation of pH in the duodenum, (4) mechanical disintegration, (5) absorption, and (6) transport. Since the generation of such motility patterns are highly variable and regulated by neurohormonal cues, the process of digestion has been a challenge, hitherto, to explore the mechanisms involved.

The mechanical relevance to digestion dates back to the classical study performed by Cannon on cat's intestine using X-ray [1]. The observations made by Cannon reports, *The constrictions causing the segmentation thoroughly mix the food and digestive juices, and bring the digested food into contact with the absorbing mechanisms* [1]. Even after a century has passed, the digestion still remains to be mystery; probably due to the multifaceted dimensions of the digestive process. In the recent past, there has been growing literature on the involvement of the mechanics in the digestion. Studies indicate that the mechanics of peristalsis is intertwined with physiological function of the intestine and still remains to be explored. The idea that the mechanics play a key role in the intestinal physiology is best described by Costa and Brookes which reads, *The discovery of the presence of multiple neurochemicals in the same nerve cells in specific combinations led to the concept of "chemical coding" and of "plurichemical transmission." The proposal that enteric reflexes are largely responsible for the propulsion of contents led to investigations of polarized reflex pathways and how these may be activated to generate the coordinated propulsive behavior of the intestine* [2]. We learn that the digestion system include highly complex organ which manages, *in house*, the enteric controls that are mediated through intramural reflexes (short and long range reflexes), and centralized control mediated through the central nervous system (involving higher nerves centers to process the information relating to gut sensing and relay through efferent nerves). While it has been a mystery for many decades as to how the digestion occurs in the gut, especially the mechanical breakdown, mixing and transiting over the long distance of the bowels, recent studies on mechanics are providing clues pertaining to the mechanisms that may contribute towards an understanding of the process involved at the level of mechanical digestion and their interaction with upstream and downstream players.

In this chapter, we present the current state of art in the area of intestinal biomechanics addressing various aspects of digestion through clinical, mathematical, and computational studies performed so far. This chapter is organized as follows: Section 2 describes the mechanics and physiology of the small intestine. Section 3 provides details as to how the small intestinal motility leads to the development of flows inside the lumen causing mixing and transport. The details of flow resulting from circular contraction are discussed in Section 4. In Section 5, the relevance of the local longitudinal shortening is explored followed by the physiological relevance of motility in Section 6. Since the nature of forces also affect the molecular biology of the cell, the basic principle behind the mechanotransduction is addressed in Section 7. The conclusions are drawn in Section 8 followed by the future scope of the work in Section 9.

2. Mechanophysiology of the small intestine and the small intestinal digestion

2.1 Anatomy

The small intestine is the part of the gastrointestinal tract which connects to the stomach at one end through pylorus and the large intestine at the other end through ileocecal valve (**Figure 1**). The anatomy of the small intestine segments, that includes duodenum, jejunum, and ileum, are discussed in the following.

2.1.1 Antrum

The antrum is a distal part of the stomach which is highly muscular having a thickness of 5.1 ± 1.6 mm (depends on degree of distention of antrum [3]), which

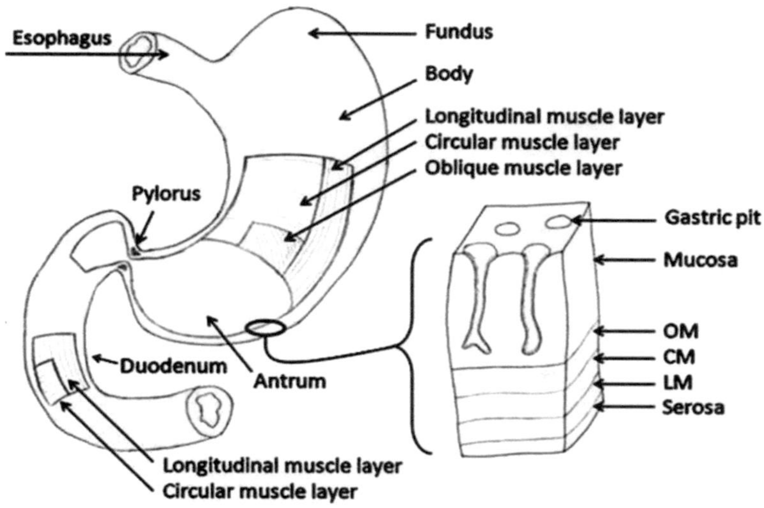

Figure 1.
Anatomical details of the stomach and duodenum showing three layers of muscles—oblique muscle layer (OM), circular muscle layer (CM), and longitudinal muscle layer (LM).

is higher than proximal stomach [4]. Its musculature helps the antral segment to undergo rigorous peristalsis to perform the grinding of the food. They also help regulating the gastric emptying and duodenogastric reflux (DGR).

2.1.2 Pylorus

The pylorus (at L1 level or Lumber region 1) is a muscular tissue that connects the stomach at one end to the small intestine or more specifically the duodenum at the other end. Due to its musculature they contract radially to close or open the valve to cause the flow across the stomach and duodenum. It functions like a valve whereby it can regulate the flow of gastric content into the duodenum.

2.1.3 Small intestine

The small intestine is a muscular and convoluted tube that extends from pyloric region to the ileocecal valve that connects to the large intestine. It is approximately 7 m long and 2–4 cm in diameters and divided into the duodenum, jejunum, and ileum.

2.1.3.1 Duodenum

Duodenum is the shortest segment of them all and is approximately 20–25 cm long and 2.5 cm in diameter. They are responsible to mix the chyme with DBP secretions, cause homogenization and pH transition from acidic to slightly alkaline. The process occurs inside the segment that is divided into four parts as follows: (1) the first part or par superior or duodenal bulb is about 5 cm long which begins its journey somewhere at the pylorus region and ends at the neck region of the gall bladder. Pars superior is the most movable region of the duodenum. (2) The second part or pars descendens is about 7–10 cm long and extends from the neck region of the gall bladder or L1 (lumbar region 1) to the upper border of L4 region. The common bile duct and the pancreatic duct together join and open at the major duodenal papilla into the medial side of this segment at approximately 7–10 cm distance from the pylorus. The minor duodenal papilla, if present, lies above the major duodenal papilla. (3) The third part or pars horizontalis is about 5–7.5 cm long and travels across the inferior vena cava and aorta above the upper border of the fourth lumbar region with the superior mesenteric vessels (the vein on the right and the artery on the left) on its front. (4) The fourth part or pars ascendens is about 2.5 cm long and continues to ascend toward the left side of the aorta. At its terminus, it abruptly transforms to a jejuna-like feature, where it forms the duodeno-jejunal flexure. The duodeno-jejunal flexure is connected to the superior mesenteric artery and celiac artery by suspensory muscles of the duodenum also known as the ligament of Treitz (a connective tissue), which marks the anatomical distinction between the duodenum and the jejunum.

2.1.3.2 Jejunum

It forms second part of the small intestine that is roughly 1.5–3.5 m (two-fifth of the small intestine) in length. They are attached to the posterior wall of the abdomen by the mesentery. The interior wall of the segment contains of numerous microscopic finger-like structures known as villi that help increase the surface area of absorption for the jejunum. Most of the nutrients are absorbed in this part of the small intestine. By the time the intestinal contents are emptied into the next segment (ileum), around 90% of all the available nutrients in the food has been absorbed. It also helps to shape the rheology of the digesta by absorbing about 90% of the secreted water, 6–8 l day^{-1}.

2.1.3.3 Ileum

It forms the last segment of the intestine that is roughly 2.5–3.5 m (three-fifth of the small intestine) in length and ends at the intraperitoneal pouch known as cecum (where undigested food settle down). The remaining parts of the nutrients that have passed through the jejunum are absorbed here (also absorbs vitamin B12 and bile acids). The segment contains numerous lymphoid follicles (forming Payer's patch; mainly function to survey and respond to pathogens). They are attached to the posterior wall of the abdomen by mesentery (giving flexibility to the bowels to adjust in the abdominal cavity during act of peristalsis and intestinal transit).

2.1.4 Ileocecal valve (ileal ostium)

The valve is a muscular tissue that separates the contents of the small intestine from those of the large intestine. They help in controlling the volume of flow occurring from the large intestine into the ileum and as a consequence of this, help in regulating the bacterial growth (involved in causing small intestinal bacterial overgrowth; SIBO) in the small intestine in conjunction with the small intestinal motility. It also helps in vitamin B12 absorption and collecting most of bile acid (terminal ileum) to replenish for the secreted bile for reuse (via entero hepatic circulation) [5]. They play a key role in preventing reflux of the bacteria-rich content from the large intestine into the small intestine; thus forming a barrier separating the two bowels.

2.2 Generation of smooth muscle contractions: the precursor to luminal flows

The intestinal musculature comprises of the smooth muscle fibers arranged in intertwined bundles; interconnected to the neighboring smooth muscle fibers through gap junctions. This enables two neighboring muscles to be electrical coupled. The gap junctions provide a way to propagate the electric potential (a wave of depolarization) from one fiber to the other, thereby spreading across adjacent segment of the intestine resulting in a muscular contraction (initiated as a consequence of depolarization above threshold) to traverse the segment. In physiology, the membrane of the small intestinal smooth muscle (especially the myogenic cells) cell shows rhythmic changes in their electric potential which is referred to as the slow waves (resting membrane potential of −50 to −60 mV). Slow waves are the waves of partial depolarization of the membrane having the transmembrane potential of 5–15 mV. They help in nominal depolarization of the membrane, but do not initiate a muscle contraction. It is only during the condition when the membrane potential of smooth muscle cell cross the threshold level, an action potential is triggered causing contraction of the smooth muscle fiber. The event of spiking is known to occur at the crests of slow waves. To initiate the spike potential, it is necessary that smooth muscles of the segment are in the charged condition; having the neurotransmitters released in the vicinity by neurons. The neurotransmitters are released in response to a variety of stimuli such as neural signaling form higher center of the brain (mediated through vagus nerve), and distention-induced signaling (locally mediated through intramural reflex).

2.3 Control of smooth muscle contractions through sensing

Before we discuss the factors affecting APD motility, it is worth considering the sensory-motor integration of the intestinal segments (**Figure 2**). Generation of motility patterns is in some way hardwired to the sensors present and it is because of this reason that the APD segment can show a wide variation in its motility patterns. Little is known about the neurohormonal control, chemical control (pH [6], osmolarity [6, 7], lipid (also ileum) [8, 9], carbohydrates, and proteins), and other factors like size of bolus [10] and allergic responses through jejunal dysmotility [11]. They control muscles in the APD segment (also present in jejunal and ileal

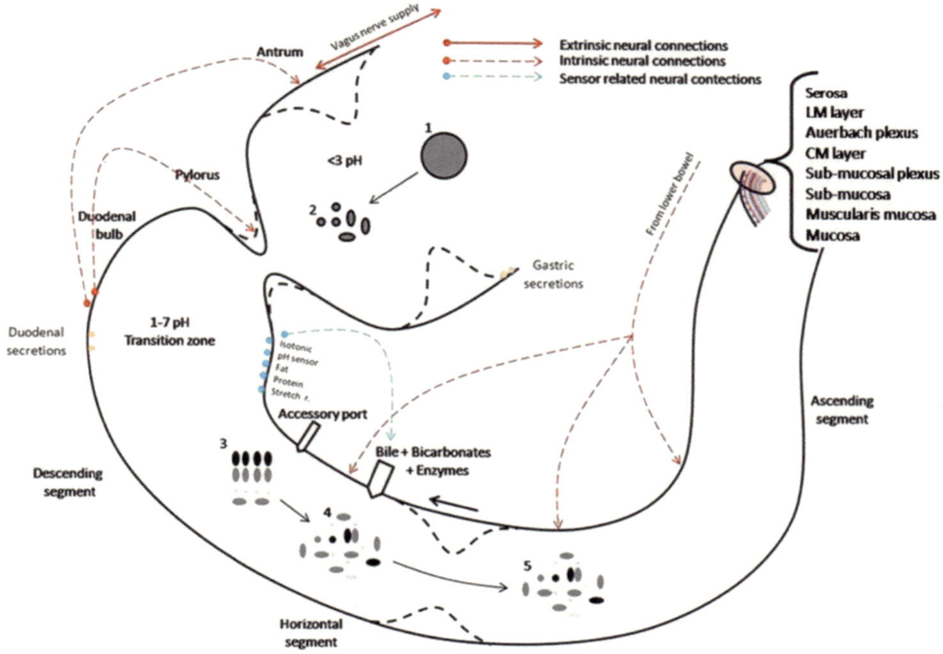

Figure 2.
A cartoon representing mechanophysiology of the APD segment; indicating (1) the bolus undergoes disintegration due to grinding activity of the stomach, (2) smaller pieces of food, (3) food in its finely disintegrated form and yet to be mixed with DBP secretions, and (4 and 5) homogeneous mixture.

segments), which help in regulation of motor patterns mediated by some kind of sensor mechanism. To support the relevance of sensory-motor integrity, let us consider the report by Peter Holzer who suggested that prevention of acid damage to the mucosal tissues are carried out by an *elaborate network of acid-governed mechanisms* that help in protecting the tissue from acidosis and maintaining homeostasis [12]. The pH distribution of the gut lumen follows a particular trend, having lowest at the stomach (pH 1–3) and then goes on increasing from duodenum (pH 1.7–5 at proximal duodenum and pH 5–6 at distal duodenum) to terminal ileum (pH 7–9) [13, 14]. On exposure of the duodenum to acidic contents they stimulate various defense mechanisms which include increase in mucosal secretions, bicarbonate secretions, and blood flow. Together with this, hormones also play a major role in acid secretion at the stomach which in turn may contribute to the overall homeostasis. The pylorus also plays its role in regulatory mechanisms which run across the terminal stomach to proximal duodenum and shares the neural tracts and the circular muscle layer with antrum and duodenum. Besides being a muscular tissue, it also has sensors embedded within its mucosal layers, which are involved in some control related activities that are relayed through enteric nervous system or local mediated reflex pathway. Digestive processes are driven by the peristalsis motion that grinds the food rigorously in the antrum, so as to grind into small pieces less than 3 mm, so that they can escape the pyloric channel. The remaining part of the digestion is driven by the intestinal peristalsis which together with chemical secretions facilitates the process of mechanical and chemical degradation of the chyme into macromolecules and further down to simpler molecules so they can be absorbed (**Figure 2**)—steps 3–5.

2.4 Coordination among the small intestinal segments

The APD contractions are very much time synchronized and work in coordination. These neurally activated contractions push the luminal contents by transferring their momentum, which helps to facilitate mixing, grinding, and transporting of the food. Two kinds of pumping action take place here, one at the antral side and the other in duodenum which tries to push their contents to the other side. It is not well understood on how these two motor actions play their part in causing the transport, i.e., either gastric emptying or reflux of duodenal content back into the stomach. However, from a mechanics point of view, we know that the flow would result in emptying when the pressure at the antral side is higher than duodenal side (**Figure 3**). However, a reverse situation can exist, i.e., reflux when duodenal pressure becomes higher than antral pressure leading to a disease condition known as the duodenogastric reflux (DGR). The mechanism by which the transport across the pylorus occurs is not clear; however, it is known that the transport occurs by developing two kinds of pressure waves via pressure pump (common cavity pressure wave) and peristaltic activity [15]. Multiple studies have been performed for estimating gastric emptying in relation to the generation of intragastric pressures using manometric studies. Though little is known about the relationship between the pump mechanism (gastric pumping) and the coordinative muscle contractions, few researchers have reported that the process of gastric emptying is observed only during those occasions when the antral pressure (Pa) is higher than the duodenal pressure (Pd). Study also indicates that the base line pressure or the common cavity pressure is the major determinant of gastric emptying (GE) rather than the antral contraction-induced emptying [15]. This idea is supported by literature which demonstrates that alternations in pressure inside the proximal stomach correlate well with the varying rates of gastric emptying of different liquid meals [16].

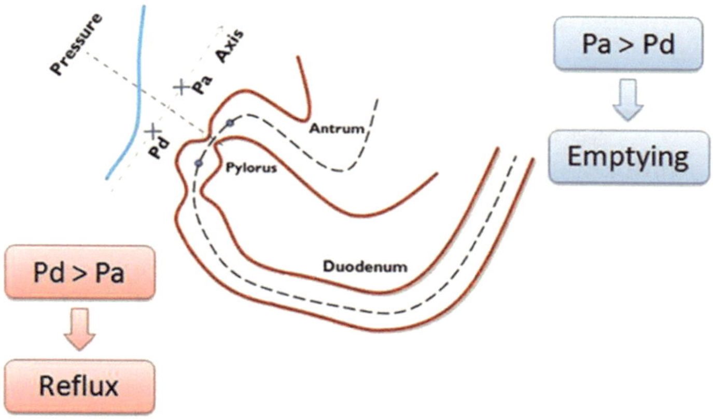

Figure 3.
A cartoon diagram depicting the antrum, pylorus, and the duodenal (APD) segments, respectively. The dashed line represents the APD axis, while the blue colored plot shows pressure profile along the axial direction indicating higher antral pressure (Pa) in comparison to lower duodenal pressure (Pd).

The local generation of high pressure and appearance of anterograde and retrograde flow patterns suggest that the geometry is closely linked to the way emptying proceeds. In addition to the complexity present in gastric emptying predictions, the gut works by intelligently sensing the food content and accordingly modulating the contraction patterns.

The coordination is established through neural feedback means; e.g., enterogastric, ileogastric, intestino-intestinal reflex, and vago-vagal reflexes. One of the well-known reflexes is the ileal brake. The ileal brake refers to the ability of the ileal segments to modulate the motility patterns upon exposure to the nutrients such as lipid through enteric reflex [17]. The intestinal segments communicate with each other through such reflex in process to regulate the digestive process such as regulating the flow at which the gastric contents enter into the duodenum by suppressing pyloric channel.

3. From small intestinal motility to flows to the digestion

A fluid is a substance which continually deforms under the application of a shear force. When an external force is applied to a solid object it undergoes whole body translation; whereas, fluid undergoes both translation and deformation. Transport of fluid can be better appreciated by considering an example of the flow through a cylindrical pipe, also referred to as the Hagen-Poiseuille flow (flow in a cylindrical pipe). Applying a relatively higher pressure force at left end of the tube, in comparison to right end, sets up a pressure gradient along the length of the tube. As a result of this, the fluid tends to move down the pressure gradient only if it has overcome the viscous resistance. In the case of viscous flow the fluid eventually gains inertia and reaches a steady state when the axial velocity profile becomes parabolic. In a similar fashion, we can draw some parallels between the Hagen-Poiseuille flows to those of intestinal flows. In physiological scenario, as the contraction (i.e., the circular constriction that appear around the periphery) propagate thorough the small intestinal segment, it imparts a part of the momentum to the fluid underneath, which as a consequence of having gained the momentum can now hit the neighboring fluid particle and transmits a part of its momentum; eventually developing the flow.

4. Mechanics of small intestinal digestion: mixing, transport, and absorption

4.1 Basic mechanics

4.1.1 Law of Laplace

We discuss the basic principles of mechanics as applied to the small intestine. The small intestine, as we know, is a muscular conduit having two types of muscle layers—circular and longitudinal muscles. When muscles undergo contraction (reduction in the length of the muscles) they happen to either close the lumen (circular contraction) or shorten the segment (longitudinal contraction). From mechanics point of view, such contraction develops forces by virtue of muscular activity. By applying basic principles of mechanics, we can deduce as to how the muscular contraction results in the generation of pressure forces and flows inside the lumen. In general, whenever the tissue undergoes contraction, we explain the principle that the reduction is caused by generation of forces per unit area or stress. Parameters of interest are the percentage reduction in the length or strain that is caused by the stress. So, there exists some relation between the stress and the strain of the material under consideration. This leads us to assess the elasticity of the material or modulus of elasticity that measures the ability of the material to resistance deformation when a stress is applied to it. The nature of resistance or wall stiffness can be visualized by referring to the stress vs. strain plots obtained by allowing the material to deform under various strains and measuring the stress. The stress-strain plot provides details relevant to the mechanical properties of the tissue.

For simple geometry such as intestine approximated as a uniform and circular cylinder, the relation between the stress and luminal pressure under the assumption of thin wall is given by Laplace's law. It says that, under equilibrium condition, the tensile stress developed in wall is proportional to the intraluminal pressure and the radius of the intestinal tube. Suggesting that if the pressure inside the intestine is increased by gas formation (fermentation), for a non-significant change in the radius to wall thickness, then there would be a corresponding increase in the tensile force of the wall.

4.1.2 Flow through the channel

Transport of fluid across narrow constriction can be better appreciated by considering a familiar example of flow through a cylindrical pipe, also referred to as the Hagen-Poiseuille flow. Applying a relatively higher pressure force at left end of the tube, in comparison to the right end, causes the fluid to move down the pressure gradient only if it has overcome the viscous resistance. In case of viscous flow, the fluid eventually gains inertia and reaches a steady state when the axial velocity profile is parabolic. Let us assume a straight channel that is static (i.e., no contractions), with occlusion at the center and applied pressure at the ends as if they were generated by the APD contractions. In steady state, the flow rate can be derived as $Q = \pi r^4 \delta P/(8\ \mu l)$, which relates the rate of flow at the outlet to the pressure difference applied to the channel. Suggesting that, the flow rate is highly sensitive to the fourth power of the channel radius and inversely proportional to the channel length.

4.1.3 Longitudinal shortening

Using high-frequency ultrasound, Nicosia et al. were able to calculate the percentage reduction in the length of the longitudinal muscles [18]. As discussed in the later section, using the principle of mass conservation, the authors were able to quantify local longitudinal shortening as the ratio of longitudinal length after contraction relative to the initial length as inversely related to the ratio of cross-sectional area of the muscle after contraction relative to the initial area; $L/L^* = 1/(A/A^*)$.

4.2 Modeling small intestinal contractions

Unlike the gastric contractions, the small intestine motility patterns are not regular. In preprandial state, the small intestine enter into the interdigestive phase showing distinct patterns of activity every 90–120 min^{-1} (also known as Migrating motor complex or MMC) which include (1) a period of quiescence with no contractions (Phase I), (2) a long period of unsynchronized contractions (Phase II), and (3) a burst of strong and regular contractions (Phase III) [19]. Of these, phase III plays an important role in sweeping the undigested food particles (left over debris) and bacteria out of the small intestine and into the large intestine. However, after meal ingestion (postprandial), the small intestine switches to a more synchronized motility patterns.

4.3 Pyloric contraction

Pylorus plays a key role in mediating the flow across the stomach and the duodenum. It does by developing higher resistance to flow through closing of the lumen. They typically open and close the lumen at intervals of 20 s [20]. Flow through the channel is driven by generating a pressure gradient across the two ends of the channel and depends on luminal diameter, degree of opening, length of canal; thus, regulating gastric emptying (GE) or duodenogastric reflux (DGR) [21–26]. Both antegrade and retrograde flow have been reported in the literature to be normal; however, when the quantity of flow in the reverse direction leads to increased volume of reflux, then it leads to DGR disease. The flow is found to be pulsatile in nature [27–34]. The pylorus exhibits both tonic and phasic contractions [35–38], which develops a pressure of 10.8 ± 4.5 mmHg at 1–4 min^{-1} rates of phasic contraction [35]. In postprandial state, pylorus opens and closes with mean diameter 5.4 ± 1.0 mm [21]. Out of 193 pyloric closure events, 133 occurred in 2 s of the antral and duodenal contraction in a study carried out in patients. The pylorus was reported to be in closed position for 55.5% of 154 isolated duodenal contractions recorded. In porcine flow, pulses happen at 11.2 ± 0.4 min^{-1} frequency and occur between subsequent pyloric pressure events with each flow lasting for 3.5 ± 0.1 s with volumes of 0.3 ± 0.01 ml being release during the stroke. They occur 2.8 ± 0.7 s before pyloric pressure event, and 2.3 ± 0.5 s before antral wall motion [39]. Meal-dependent effects of pyloric motility using clinical trials of intravenous injection of 20% dextrose solution indicated causation of pyloric contraction, suppression of antral contraction, and duodenal phase-3-like motility [40]. The duration and intensity of phasic and tonic contraction of the pylorus showed direct correlation with caloric content of dextrose solution been infused into duodenum. Increase in caloric content caused increase in isolated pyloric pressure waves and basal pyloric pressure [41]. Duodenal infusion of saline shows no change in motility patterns of APD; whereas, triglyceride and fatty acid infusion suppresses antral contractions, but enhances pyloric phasic and tonic activity and delays gastric emptying [42, 43].

4.4 Intestinal peristalsis

Contractions of the intestine are a mix of elementary contractions such as stationary (SW), antegrade (APW), or retrograde propagating wave (RPW). A literature survey of the motility patterns indicate frequency of 15–18 wave min^{-1}, velocity of propagation of 0.1–0.4 cm s^{-1}, and higher propensity to develop propagating contraction in the intestine in comparison to stationary contraction [44]. Retroperistalsis have been linked to the reflux of duodenal contents and trigger the development of DGR diseases. Standing contractions are the non-propagating contractions they are confined over a particular segment (12 waves min^{-1}). They are known to be involved in the mixing process. Contractions appearing on one side of the channel are known as sleeve contractions. It involves longitudinal muscle for generating contraction [45] and help in mixing and churning of luminal contents [46]. Pendular movements are the longitudinal contraction of the muscles, which develops motility patterns involving to-and-fro motions of segmental shortening and extension. In physiology, the contractions occur as a mixture of the basic contractions, as discussed above. It is a well-known fact that upon nutrient infusion of duodenum, the duodenal motility patterns changes from propulsive to a segmental contraction that traveled only for a short span. Such contractions form segmental contractions or cluster contractions, which can be stationary or non-stationary [47].

4.5 Flow due to circular muscle contractions

Flow due to circular contraction were investigated by the author by approximating the flow for a Newtonian liquid meal with viscosity 1000 cP and density 1000 g cc^{-1} inside the APD segment [44]. The rationale for choosing such an assumption was—(1) for a liquid meal intake the meal mixes with gastric and duodeno-biliary-pancreatic secretions giving a mixture that is also a liquid; (2) the rheology of the contents present inside the duodenum is not yet known; therefore, a Newtonian approximation was made; (3) modeling a semi-solid meal increases the complexity, therefore, a liquid meal was considered to simplify the development of the APD segment. Further, the APD segment was assumed to be a rigid wall to simplify the flow model.

There is a formation of recirculation eddies near the occlusion zone (with velocities reaching its peak at its center) and occurrence of a local transport at the pyloric region (arising due to the pressure difference across it) (**Figure 4**). Results indicate that a retrograde moving wave cause pressurization at the head region of the wave in comparison to the tail region. As a result of this behavior, a steep pressure rise is developed to cause flow in the direction that is downward the steep. It was also found that this wave generates a pressure difference across the pylorus, that is, higher pressure on the antrum side in comparison to a lower pressure on proximal duodenum thereby causing reflux.

To understand the impact of variations in the intestinal peristalsis, the author performed a parametric study by varying the geometry and wave parameters of the contraction. Based on literature, a hypothetical range was considered for these parameters presuming that this range falls within the physiological regime.

The study demonstrated that higher degrees of occlusion and higher velocity for the propagatory contractions have a profound effect on the flow rate across the channel (**Table 1**). Although, for APWs, the emptying rate increases with occurrence of multiple waves, they also induce reflux when occurring in four numbers spread across the duodenum and centered at 8 cm away from pylorus. The effect of multiplicity in the RPW shows an increasing trend in reflux. In general, it can be interpreted that the APW type contractions lead to emptying while RPW lead to reflux.

Standing contractions (SW type) of closing type were found to be reflux inducing. However, they occur at less than one-tenth of a magnitude for variations in distance, wavelength, and degree of occlusion in comparison to the APW and the RPW contractions. They also show an increasing level of reflux with increasing values of parameters except for distance. When multiple standing waves occur they result in significant increase in the reflux.

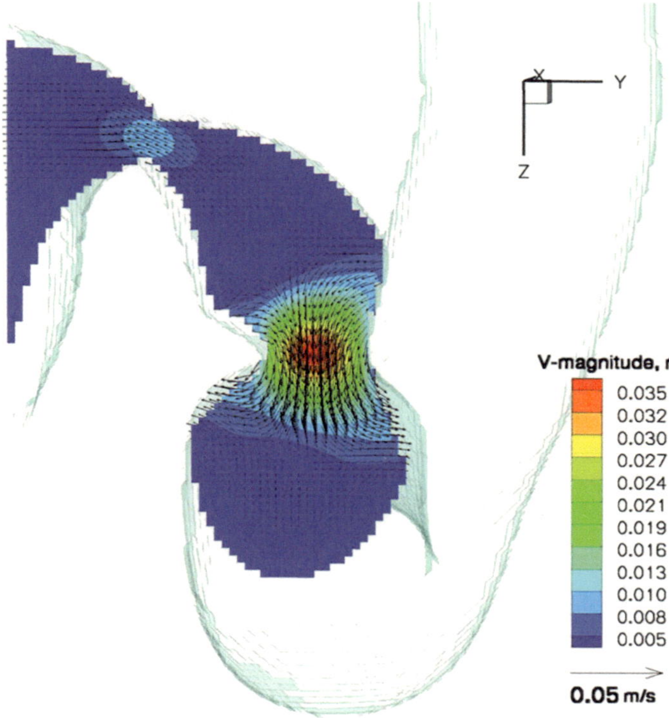

Figure 4.
Flow due retrograde wave traveling toward the pylorus. Arrows indicate velocity vector over the local region and colors indicate the magnitude.

On overall comparison of the reflux levels caused by the elementary contractions, it is clear that the SW of higher frequency and the RPW of higher occlusion (70%), higher velocity and occurring in multiple numbers dominate the list of reflux inducing contractions of the duodenum.

The APW and RPW contraction show mixing at higher intensity that is typically of the order of hundreds that is ten times those of SW. Variations in distance and wavelengths of the APW and RPW type contractions show similar levels of mixing (**Table 2**). Contractions cause higher degree of mixing with increasing occlusions and are highly sensitive to the velocity, wherein a change from 1 to 4 cm s^{-1} can lead to a ten-fold increase in I_{mixing}. Further, it was seen that multiple waves can cause significant rise in mixing. However, the standing contractions show negligible mixing that are typically of the order of tens and are highly sensitive to frequency and multiple waves. While I_{mixing} shows extent of mixing in the whole duodenum,

Contraction type	Distance (↑)	Wavelength (↑)	% Occlusion (↑)	Velocity (cm s^{-1}) or frequency (↑)	Multiple waves (↑)
APW	Negligible	Negligible	↑	↑	↑
RPW	Negligible	Negligible	↑	↑	↑
SW*	↓	↑	↑	↑	↑

**For SW, frequency is considered. APW, antegrade propagating wave; RPW, retrograde propagating wave; and SW, standing wave.*

Table 1.
Effects of duodenal pumping on transpyloric flow rate (GE or DGR) studied for various parameters of APW, RPW, and SW type of contractions.

Contraction type	Distance (↑)	Wavelength (↑)	% Occlusion (↑)	Velocity (cm s^{-1}) or frequency (↑)	Multiple waves (↑)
APW	↑ or ↓	↓	↑	↑	↑ or ↓
RPW	Negligible	↑	↑	↑	↑
SW	↓	↑	↑	↑	↑

Table 2.
Effect of APD contractions on intensity of mixing.

Contraction type	Distance (↑)	Wavelength (↑)	% occlusion (↑)	Velocity (cm s^{-1}) or frequency (↑)	Multiple waves (↑)
APW	Negligible	Negligible	↑	↑	↑
RPW	Negligible	Negligible	↑	↑	↑
SW	Negligible	Negligible	Negligible	↑	Negligible

Table 3.
Effect of APD contractions on volume of mixing.

we also wanted to quantify the region over which the mixing or the volume of mixing is significant (computed as the volume of duodenum that has mixing index above 1.005). Changes in distance and wavelength of the peristaltic waves showed no major change in volume of mixing; however, it was sensitive to occlusion to some extent and highly sensitive to velocity and multiple waves. Standing contractions, on the other hand, showed zero or negligible volumes of mixing, except for a frequency of 6 Hz where they showed some mixing (**Table 3**).

5. Significance of the longitudinal muscles

5.1 What is LLS?

Contractions of the longitudinal muscles, when occurring over short range of the gut segment, are referred to as the local longitudinal shortening. In literature, longitudinal shortening have been investigated as if they are advancing with the contraction, which we define as the advancing LLS and those that are stationary or stationary LLS are rarely considered. During LLS, the longitudinal muscles contract to shorten the segment along the axial direction only.

5.2 Learning from esophageal studies of LLS

LLS studies of the intestinal segments have been rarely considered. In order to understand the mechanophysiology of the LLS in intestine, we resort to the LLS studies of the esophageal segment.

One of the classical studies of LLS was the study of esophageal peristalsis during feline. By using a widely spaced metal clips clamped to the esophageal mucosa (four tantalum wires that were imbedded in the outer esophageal wall), Dodds et al. [48] captured the longitudinal shortening of the esophageal segment which varies with their relative position. The study demonstrated the existence of a wave of local longitudinal shortening that moves in conjunction with the bolus. They also found that the relative displacements of the markers vary from one location to the other location suggesting that the LLS is effective over a given segment of the esophagus (especially the distal most esophagus). Subsequent studies, using widely spaced metal clips attached to the esophageal mucosa, support the contractive nature of the longitudinal muscles in the local regions of the esophageal wall during peristalsis [49–51]. Measuring local longitudinal shortening was, however, a challenge using the mucosal clip studies; given the large spacing of 3–10 cm. Nicosia et al. provided a more accurate method of determining the LLS and their coordination with CC using the high-frequency ultrasound transducer [18]. By employing the principle of law of mass conservation, the changes in the cross-sectional area with the temporal variation in local longitudinal shortening was made; which were compared with the luminal pressure measured using high resolution manometry. Following relation was derived: cross-sectional area during rest phase/cross-sectional area during contraction = length of the segment during contracted state/length during rest. Key observations were as follows: (1) during luminal filling (with bolus entry), the esophagus distends reducing the effective thickness of the muscles, (2) the wave of longitudinal shortening was followed by the circular contraction, (3) contraction of the longitudinal muscles were found to nearly coincide with the peak luminal pressure, (4) longitudinal shortening overlaps the CC and occur prior to CC and ended after CC, and (5) lastly, the strength of LLS directly relates to the generation of higher luminal pressure. Further clinical studies by the investigators also indicate the prior contraction of the longitudinal muscle during onset of distal esophageal peristalasis [18, 49, 50]. Such fine coordination the contraction of two muscles fibers provides for a mechanical advantage of gathering the neighboring circular muscle fiber closer to ensure that the circular contraction occurs at ease [52]. The coordination of CC and LLS is managed by the enteric and central nervous system. The delay in the onset of contraction is due to the existence of a gradient of latency of contraction along the length of the esophagus [53].

5.3 Effect of advancing LLS on flows

Like the peristalsis waves (which are modeling as trains of periodic sinusoidal waves traversing the muscular tube at certain velocity), the LLS is modeled as a sinusoidal wave whose amplitude relates to the local shortening (l/l_0) and propagates with the CC. As shown in **Figure 5**, LLS brings together the neighboring tissues through generation of a localized wave of shortening. As a result of this, the circular muscles become denser giving its advantage to compress the lumen at ease. We consider that the longitudinal contraction is in relative motion to the CC; hence, we define them as LLS of advancing type.

As the LLS traverse the intestine with CC, the intestinal wall undergoes deformation. Such change in the wall generates wall momentum which acts as a source of energy to push the fluid and develop flows. The details of the wall motions are provided in the form of a local wall velocity in **Figure 5**. Circular contractions are wall motions that appear as ripples traveling over the surface of water. As the circular muscles contract, the wall moves radially inward; however, as the wave moves at certain velocity they appear to close the head region of the wave leaving behind the tail end to relax or open (outward velocity vector; first panel in **Figure 5**). For advancing LLS, a wave of localized shortening occurs which travels at certain speed. During such activity, the surface of the intestinal wall appear to move forward but recoils back to its original position after the disturbance has traverse the segment. This generates a net forward velocity, as shown in second panel of **Figure 5**. Superimposing both the waves result in a summation of the two velocity vectors (third panel in **Figure 5**). We may summarize that the introduction of LLS results in an axial displacement of the wall and CC in radial displacement.

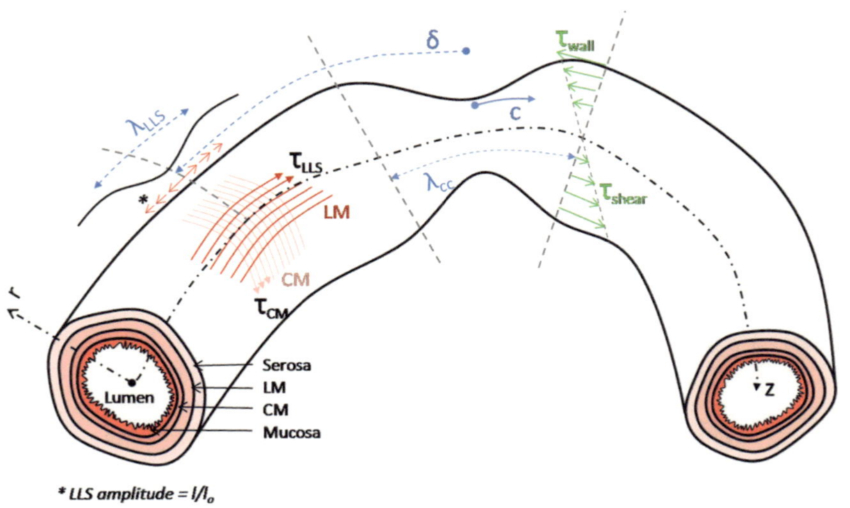

Figure 5.
A cartoon diagram illustrating the circular (CC) and longitudinal contractions (LLS) in the intestinal wall. L is the length and R is the radius of the intestine. CC is characterized by the wavelength (λ) and the percentage occlusion of the lumen (p_{occ}). Peak value of LLS is given by the peak l/lo ratio which is spaced at a relative distance (δ) from the peak CC or the point of maximal occlusion.

Considering no-slip condition (fluid particle at wall moves with the same velocity with which the wall moves), we also learn that there is an effective axial displacement of the fluid adjacent to wall and helps to drag the peripheral part of the food along with it (**Figure 6**).

Rheology plays an essential role in regulating the transport of the digesta from stomach to duodenum (gastric emptying) and duodenum (duodenogastric reflux). For a meal that is highly viscous, the mixing and transport can be a difficult task to be performed by the enteric system when compared to low viscous digesta. Since the mechanical processes taking part in intestine correlates to the rate at which absorption takes place and determines the serum glucose levels, the subject matter is of high relevance to satiety, indigestion, and other digestive disorders of the gut.

Let us estimate the flow regime of water, juice, and honey. We consider an intestinal geometry with diameter 2.5 cm (2.5–3 cm), and wave traveling at a characteristic velocity of 2.5 cm s^{-1} (2.5–5 cm s^{-1}) for short and long wavelength of one and ten times the diameter. Assuming a fluid density of 1 g cc^{-1} and fluid viscosities of 1 cP (water), 0.65P (juice), and 33P (honey) and substituting into the formula ($Re = \rho v D/\mu$) we determine Reynolds number as 625, 9.615, and 0.189. As per the long wavelength approximation [54], we perform viscous scaling by a factor (=diameter/wavelength of the wave) to get an approximate Reynolds number. At one-tenth of scaling, the Reynolds number is found to be 62.5, 0.9615, and 0.0189. At higher Reynolds number, the inertial forces of the fluid are much higher than viscous resistance and as a result lead to turbulence flow. We speculate that a fast moving contraction of the intestine help in pushing the fluid to a higher extent that it leads to turbulence and upon interaction with air leads to borborygmus (a rumbling, growling or gurgling noise of the intestine). The studies of the bowel sounds (auscultation) were pioneered by Cannon in the early twentieth century. However, due to technical challenges, the method appears to be of some hope to clinicians in diagnosing GI disorders through bowel sound computational analysis (BSCA) [55]. At low *Re*, the flows are laminar and silent.

Flow details of the intestinal peristalsis have been recently reported in the literature [56]. When a wave of contraction propagates along the intestinal wall, they develop peripheral forces that can be directed radially inward, axially oriented,

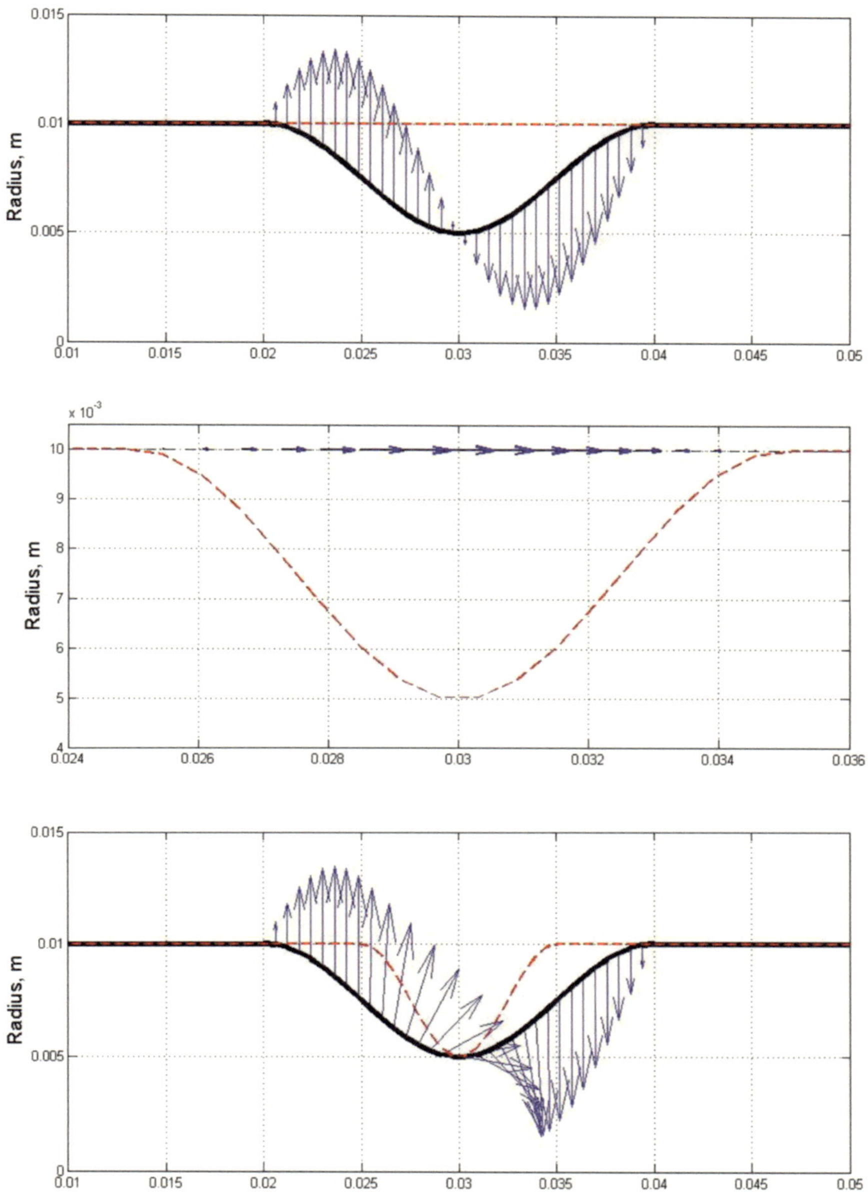

Figure 6.
A snapshot of a simulation study indicating the wall velocity (blue line) along the radial direction (CC) and no shortening (LLS, red line) (first panel). Study involving LLS (approximated by sinusoidal waveform) without CC; the wall is pulled toward the point of peak LLS (second panel). Effect of CC and LLS on wall velocity.

or inclined depending on the nature of contraction (CC and/or LLS) (**Figure 7**). As a result, the head region develops a higher pressure relative to the tail end. While at the tail end, development of low pressure field results from the retraction of the wall as if they were to open the channel. As a result the development of differential pressure forces across the segment, a pressure gradient which acts as a driving force to propel the luminal contents from a region of higher pressure to the lower pressure (retrograde flow). Flow due to advancing LLS is less prominent due to generation of low fluid velocity and low shear stress. Since they develop axial velocity at the wall, the advancing LLS, through viscous behavior, drags the neighboring fluid to move along with the wall creating a whirlpool-like motion in the region of contraction.

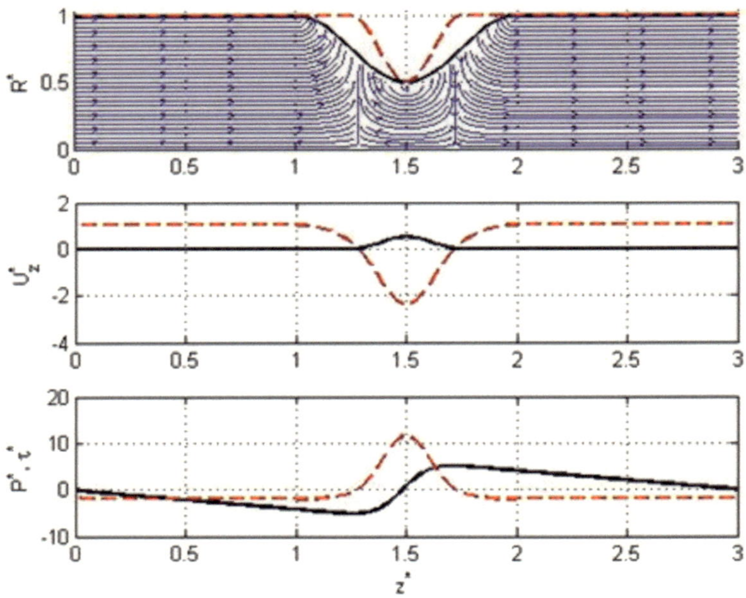

Figure 7.
Effect of simultaneous circular and longitudinal contractions on flow.

The advancing LLS and CC lead to the generation of pressure field and shear stress of similar trend. Local variations in the pressure along the axis indicate a linear variation in the non-contraction region and a nonlinear variation in the contraction region; zero at the center and boundaries—inlet and outlet of the intestinal segment. The pressure peaks at an offset from the center and shows symmetry about the axis for a contraction wave at the mid-segment. The wall shear stress shows a peak at the center of the contraction region and reduces to lower value at the either end of the wave and remains constant throughout the non-contraction region. Axial variations in the pressure and wall shear stress are similar for fluid of pseudo-plastic, Newtonian, and dilatants type. The study also reports that the pressure developed is higher for shear thickening fluids in comparison to shear-thinning fluid (**Table 4**). In a similar manner, wall shearing is highest for the dilatants. Shear stress in the lumen is highest at the wall and reduces linearly to the lowest value

Parameter (↑)	Pressure	Shear stress	Flow rate	Peak luminal velocity	Physiological relevance
Viscosity	↑	↑	No change	No change	Extent of viscous behavior
Flow behavior index	↑	↑	↓	↓	Captures the rheology of diverse fluids
LLS spacing (about optimal)	↓	↓	↑ or ↓	↑ or ↓	CC and LLS coordination
Wavelength	↑ or ↓	↓	↑	↑	Effect of motility
Occlusion	↑	↑	↑	↑	Effect of motility

Table 4.
Effect of contractility and rheology (normalized values) on flow; based on semi-analytical method.

at the center. At region where the shearing is higher there is a more stirring of the fluid. CC and LLS coordination is found to affect the luminal pressure, shearing of the contents, flow rate, and peak velocity significantly.

6. Physiological relevance of intestinal motility

6.1 Mixing

Using imaginary tracers, the author was able to determine particle trajectories due to the peristalsis—CC and LLS [56]. Two kinds of flows were observed; one resulting in axial displacement of the fluid and other causing circulation of the fluids (eddies). The radial displacement brought the fluid from the core region to the periphery and vice versa; thus allowing for flushing of the fluid proximal to the mucosa. However, the particles were displaced when the wave traverses the segment. Particle motion is highly dependent on the type of intestinal motility. Positioning of the tracers at various depths of the lumen showed different trajectory and followed the wall; particles close to the wall tend to follow the wall, while those near the axis exhibited near circulation. The authors report that the radial dimension of the whorls is found to be higher when the particles were positioned close to the wall and least at the center. Suggesting that, the contractions are more effective near the wall since the particles experience most of the wall momentum and least at the center of the lumen. Such a behavior is indicative of the mixing of the contents; given that the shearing is effective near the wall with formation of eddies.

6.2 Transport

When contraction traverses at 50% occlusion, there is a higher tendency for the particles to undergo circulation; favoring mixing [56]. However, at 80% occlusion, the particles tend to under more of axial displacement and less of a radial displacement with no circulation; favoring transport. Particles positioned near the center were found to travel a longer distance in comparison to those near the wall. Such behavior reminds us the parabolic velocity profile in case of pressure driven flows in pipe. Previous studies corroborates with the understanding that the flows in occlusion regions tend to show a parabolic profile [44]. Rheological effects of the particle displacement suggest that the eccentricity of the particle trajectory for Newtonian fluid is more and undergoes a near complete circulation. Particle trajectory for dilatants showed formation of a complete circulation. For fluid having flow behavior index less than 1.0, following observations were made (1) particles tend to travel with higher velocity over longer distance and (2) particles showed more of a radial predominance. There were no significant changes in the flow developed by introducing the LLS; however, due to additional momentum along the axial direction they tend to suppress the radial displacement of the tracer leading to a more translocation. The transport has been linked to malabsorption of the nutrients and electrolyte concentration. Alternations in the intestinal transit can disturb the equilibrium of osmolality and intestinal absorption leading to diarrhea or constipation [57]. Knowledge of the intestinal transit of bolus is essential when design the drug. Orally administered drugs have to be tuned to the environmental conditions of the small intestine so that drug bioavailability can be maximized. Since the physical properties of the meal, such as viscosity can greatly influence the transport behavior, clinical preparation of the food can be administered to help manage the patient suffering from motility disorders.

6.3 Frictional advantage

Frictional effects of the intestinal wall have been attributed to a disadvantage when considering transport. By estimating the flow resistance, the author was able to assess the importance of the slowing down of the fluid flow and increase in the retention time of the fluid near the mucosa; providing more time to undergo chemical digestion and absorption [56]. The extent of friction offered by the intestine to fluid of different flow behavior index (n = 0.6, 1.0, and 1.4) suggests that the friction is highest for pseudo-plastics and decreases with increase in flow behavior index [56]. In addition to this, friction is found to be dependent on pressure gradient; showing increasing trend with increase in pressure. They are linearly related to the Reynolds number; higher the *Re* higher is the resistance. Since the friction is analyzed for a channel with smooth inner surface, we presume that the contribution resulting from plicae circulares would be much higher.

Friction is more at the occlusion center and drops significantly as one recedes away from occlusion center to the wave end. The friction due to mucosal layer of the intestine is a subject matter of interest to intestinal digestion. We may consider the problem similar to the flooding of the terrain occupied by numerous trees. At the flood end, where the fluid velocity is very high, the fluid particles tend to slow down upon interacting with the tree. Since the surface area of the tree is more, the effectiveness to slow the fluid particle is much higher. In physiology, such resistance to flow is provided by the intestinal folds of mucosa known as the plicae circulares or the valves of kerckring. The author speculates that these structures help in reducing the luminal transport and increase the time of retention of the fluid near the mucosa so as to allow for increased absorption of the nutrients. Depending on the flow regime, the flow may be highly agitated to flush the contents and allow for replenishment of the nutrient-rich contents. Such a behavior prevents the formation of trapped fluids and cause continuous flushing of the mucosa without stagnation. Such understanding is necessary to know the dynamics of nutrient transport near the intestinal mucosa and equilibration. While, stagnation of the acidic contents near the duodenum can have drastic impact on the mucosal layer leading to duodena ulceration.

6.4 Power demands of peristalsis

Contraction leading to flow is majorly determined by the muscular contractions of the circular and longitudinal muscle layers of the intestine. Although extramural pressure forces may contribute in the modulating the flow patterns, much of the mechanics is initiated and driven by the muscles. Efficiency to pump is defined as the ratio of energy due to pressure force to the energy spent by intestine through muscular contraction. The circular contractions are majorly known to cause the positive displacement of the fluid, and hence primarily responsible to transport. However, the LLS results in the developed for axial forces that are small in comparison to circular contraction and have minor contribution to efficiency at lower occlusions. LLS is advantageous at higher occlusion, where they primarily help to forcefully shrink the intestinal wall along the axial direction to concentrate more circular fibers. The energy spent on contraction can be reduce dramatically from 26.5 (CC along) to 22.5 units (CC with 0.65% LLS) approximately; a 15% reduction in energy spent by the intestinal motility to drive shear thickening fluid. However, in contrast to the above, we also identify that power advantage of LLS negatively correlates for shear-thinning fluid driven by CC with 0.65% LLS. Suggesting that rheology of the luminal contents shares some relation with the nature of LLS. This emphasizes an important observation as to whether such a correlation exists, and if so, how does the intestine senses the fluid rheology? Although there are no direct sensors to detect the rheology or viscosity of the contents, we speculate that the gut may use an indirect mechanism to serve the purpose of assessing the rheology through stretch sensors. Since this sensor respond to distension, we also speculate that the difficulty to pump highly viscous fluid are reflected in the form of stretch. The concept of mechanical sensing of the stretch in the intestinal wall was observed by infusing a larger bolus of isotonic saline directly into the intestinal lumen [58]. The study reported that a controlled distension of the intestine activates a subset of vagal sensory neurons. Perhaps, the sensors data are relayed to the higher centers of the brain or through the local reflex to trigger certain feedback controls. Somehow, the intestine is aware of the trade-offs between the power demands of peristalsis at a certain occlusion against the percentage LLS. It may not prefer to contract at higher LLS for circular contraction of lower occlusion; since it would be non-economical. However, on the contrary, it is economical to contract at higher LLS for circular contraction of higher occlusion; an optimal strategy in conserving the amount of energy it spends to perform the peristalsis.

6.5 What is the optimal parameter space for contractility?

The intestine has its own ability to perform muscular contraction to an extent that can be mapped onto a phase space (multidimensional space in which each state variable represented by an axis is constructed to specify the state of a physical system at a given point of time). To derive such plots for intestine, we resorted to literature reports related to the clinical observations of the intestinal motility during fed and fasted state, and, normal and pathology condition [22]. The parameters of interest are: incidence of propagatory versus stationary contractions per min, percentage incidence of antegrade and retrograde propagating waves, frequency of the wave, wave velocity in mm/s, and duration of MMC (interdigestive contractions) cycle. The ability of the intestine to perform digestion optimally depends on how well it coordinates with neurohormonal system. Eliciting segmental contraction on duodenal infusion of fat or hydrochloric acid requires that the contents are mixed well with the biliopancreatic secretions to cause buffering and emulsification. Such motility patterns are known to transform the fat into droplets which help providing more surface area for lipase binding to take place and perform the digestion [59]. Previous study by the author shows intestinal preference to digestion especially extent of mixing, and volume of mixing, and to-and-fro motion of contents [44]. Since the peristalsis provides sufficient shearing forces to help cause the droplet formation, we learn that some correlation exist between the motility and emulsification. Similarly, transport of the contents requires forceful expulsion of the contents by through muscular contraction of the intestinal wall; which demands generation of sufficient forces or right motility patterns. Studies indicate that the intestine utilizes the LLS at its advantage to perform forceful contractions; with peak LLS not exceeding 65% [18, 52]. The optimal choice of wavelength at which the shearing attains its maximum value is equal to the intestinal diameter (1 unit); higher wavelength (1.5 units) is inefficient [56]. Similarly occlusive contractions show two functions—mixing at lower occlusion and transport at higher occlusion. The choice of occlusion is dependent on whether the meal needs further processing or not.

7. From wall shear and strain to influencing cell biology of the intestine

As a result of the mechanical forces arising from muscular contraction (CC, LLS, due to muscularis mucosa) or due to luminal contents (distension during gasification), the intestinal tissues are remodeled in accordance to the nature of forces. The epithelial and non-epithelial cells undergo various types of mechanical forces during the physiology function. Contractions of the circular muscle leads to generation of a tangential force along the periphery (shear) and contraction of longitudinal muscle layer leads to axial force (shear). In reality, such contractions are highly irregular and occur in conjunction that varies in wave geometry and kinetics (velocity). Shear forces at the mucosal layer affect the villi structure which modulates the adsorptive function of the organ and strain in the intramural structure affect the tissue (intestinal wall) and its compliance. The responsive nature of the intestine comes from the fact that the intestinal walls have several mechanosensitive cell types that respond to various types of mechanical stimuli such as—epithelial enterochromaffin cells (ECL), enteric neuronal cells (intrinsic and extrinsic), smooth muscle cells, and interstitial cells of Cajal (ICC). These cells contain ion channels (stretch-activated ion channel) that respond to mechanical forces and in response to stimuli they generate ionic currents in the channel thereby affecting mechanotransduction process. In mechanotransduction, the mechanical forces such as shear, stretch, and pressure trigger a biochemical pathway (through conformation change) initiating the chain reaction (involving second messengers) to affect the gene expression, and protein synthesis. *In vitro* experiment involving the seeding of scaffolds with human umbilical vein endothelial cells (HUVECs) demonstrated that the mechanical stimuli provided in the form of a pulsatile shear stress (12 ± 4 dyne cm^{-2}) leads to changes in the expression of the mechanosensitive genes (Pecam1, Enos) [60].

8. Conclusion

The digestive process of the intestine is complex and depends on multiple parameters such as rheology of food, chemical composition, motility pattern, and neurohormonal signaling. In this chapter, we have addressed the question as to how the mechanics play a key role in performing the disintegration of the partially digested food through shearing action of the peristalsis. Both circular and longitudinal contraction participate in the process in a way to optimally perform the digestion at ease; which otherwise would be uneconomical. LLS is advantageous when driving contents having shear thickening behavior, where the longitudinal shortening brings the circular muscles closer to reduce the tension in the individual fibers during peristalsis. LLS have no significant contribution in the development of the flows. In conclusion, biomechanical studies indicate that the flow is highly sensitive to the motility patterns (geometry and wave parameters), and in order to perform the digestion, the intestine elicits the right kinds of contraction to perform the physiological functions (such as preventing duodenal ulceration through segmental contraction, buffering of chyme in the duodenum, preventing duodenogastric reflux, and digestion of meal).

9. Future scope

Previous study involving the 3D computer simulations of the flow provided details of relevance to physiology. Contraction types analyzed so far include: (1) stationary contractions (contractions that close and open at a given location) (a) closure type, (b) Opening type*, (c) multiple contractions, (d) cluster/repetitive contractions; (2) propulsive contractions (contractions moving in either direction) (a) antegrade type, (b) retrograde type, (c) multiple contractions, (d) short distance traveling contractions*, (e) long distance traveling contractions*; and (3)

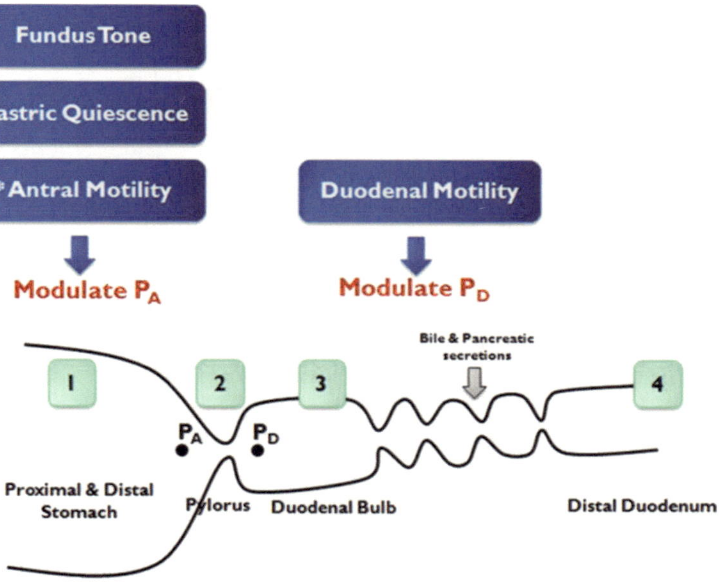

Figure 8.
Compartment model of the APD segment showing various segments (1) stomach, (2) pylorus, (3) duodenal bulb, and (4) distal duodenum.

mixed (mixture of both stationary and propulsive contractions)*. The contractions marked with * could not be analyzed due to computational limitations. This gives us a huge opportunity to the biomechanical engineers to explore the mechanism as to how the motility leads to digestion. Literature suggests a compartmental model to describe the physiological relevance of antrum, pylorus and the duodenum (**Figure 8**). The jejunal and ileal segments still remain a mystery as to how they coordinate with each other and how they contribute to digestion.

Conflict of interest

There are no conflicts of interest.

Author details

Ravi Kant Avvari
Sasi Institute of Technology and Engineering, Tadepalligudem, Andhra Pradesh, India

*Address all correspondence to: ravikant.iitk@gmail.com

References

[1] Cannon WB. The movements of the intestines studied by means of the Rontgen rays. The Journal of Medical Research. 1902;7:72-75

[2] Costa M, Brookes SH. Architecture of enteric neural circuits involved in intestinal motility. European Review for Medical and Pharmacological Sciences. 2008;**12**(Suppl 1):3-19

[3] Tongdee R, Kongkaw L, Tongdee T. A study of wall thickness of gastric antrum: Comparison among normal, benign and malignant gastric conditions on MDCT scan. Journal of the Medical Association of Thailand (Chotmaihet thangphaet). 2012;**95**:1441-1448

[4] Pickhardt PJ, Asher DB. Wall thickening of the gastric antrum as a normal finding: Multidetector CT with cadaveric comparison. AJR American Journal of Roentgenology. 2003;**181**:973-979

[5] Dawson PA, Karpen SJ. Intestinal transport and metabolism of bile acids. Journal of Lipid Research. 2015;**56**:1085-1099

[6] Rao SS, Safadi R, Lu C, Schulze-Delrieu K. Manometric responses of human duodenum during infusion of HCl, hyperosmolar saline, bile and oleic acid. Neurogastroenterology and Motility: The Official Journal of the European Gastrointestinal Motility Society. 1996;**8**:35-43

[7] Thompson DG, Wingate DL. Effects of osmoreceptor stimulation on human duodenal motor activity. Gut. 1988;**29**:173-180

[8] Spiller RC, Trotman IF, Higgins BE, Ghatei MA, Grimble GK, Lee YC, et al. The ileal brake-inhibition of jejunal motility after ileal fat perfusion in man. Gut. 1984;**25**:365-374

[9] Welch IM, Cunningham KM, Read NW. Regulation of gastric emptying by ileal nutrients in humans. Gastroenterology. 1988;**94**:401-404

[10] Dooley CP, Valenzuela JE. Duodenal volume and osmoreceptors in the stimulation of human pancreatic secretion. Gastroenterology. 1984;**86**:23-27

[11] Valeur J, Lappalainen J, Rita H, Lin AH, Kovanen PT, Berstad A, et al. Food allergy alters jejunal circular muscle contractility and induces local inflammatory cytokine expression in a mouse model. BMC Gastroenterology. 2009;**9**:33

[12] Holzer P. Taste receptors in the gastrointestinal tract. V. Acid sensing in the gastrointestinal tract. American Journal of Physiology. Gastrointestinal and Liver Physiology. 2007;**292**:G699-G705

[13] Nugent SG, Kumar D, Rampton DS, Evans DF. Intestinal luminal pH in inflammatory bowel disease: Possible determinants and implications for therapy with aminosalicylates and other drugs. Gut. 2001;**48**:571-577

[14] Fallingborg J. Intraluminal pH of the human gastrointestinal tract. Danish Medical Bulletin. 1999;**46**:183-196

[15] Indireshkumar K, Brasseur JG, Faas H, Hebbard GS, Kunz P, Dent J, et al. Relative contributions of "pressure pump" and "peristaltic pump" to gastric emptying. American Journal of Physiology. Gastrointestinal and Liver Physiology. 2000;**278**:G604-G616

[16] Hausken T, Mundt M, Samsom M. Low antroduodenal pressure gradients are responsible for gastric emptying of a low-caloric liquid meal in humans. Neurogastroenterology and Motility: The Official Journal of the European

Gastrointestinal Motility Society. 2002;**14**:97-105

[17] van Avesaat M, Troost FJ, Ripken D, Hendriks HF, Masclee AA. Ileal brake activation: Macronutrient-specific effects on eating behavior? International Journal of Obesity. 2015;**39**:235-243

[18] Nicosia MA, Brasseur JG, Liu JB, Miller LS. Local longitudinal muscle shortening of the human esophagus from high-frequency ultrasonography. American Journal of Physiology. Gastrointestinal and Liver Physiology. 2001;**281**:G1022-G1033

[19] Castedal M, Abrahamsson H. High-resolution analysis of the duodenal interdigestive phase III in humans. Neurogastroenterology and Motility. 2001;**13**:473-481

[20] Eyre-Brook IA, Smallwood RH, Linhardt GE 2nd, Johnson AG. Timing of pyloric closure in man. Studies with impedance electrodes. Digestive Diseases and Sciences. 1983;**28**:1106-1115

[21] Ehrlein HJ. Motility of the pyloric sphincter studied by the inductograph method in conscious dogs. The American Journal of Physiology. 1988;**254**:G650-G657

[22] Hinder RA. Individual and combined roles of the pylorus and the antrum in the canine gastric emptying of a liquid and a digestible solid. Gastroenterology. 1983;**84**:281-286

[23] Meyer JH, Thomson JB, Cohen MB, Shadchehr A, Mandiola SA. Sieving of solid food by the canine stomach and sieving after gastric surgery. Gastroenterology. 1979;**76**:804-813

[24] Miller J, Kauffman G, Elashoff J, Ohashi H, Carter D, Meyer JH. Search for resistances controlling canine gastric emptying of liquid meals. The American Journal of Physiology. 1981;**241**:G403-G415

[25] Schulze-Delrieu K, Brown CK. Emptying of saline meals by the cat stomach as a function of pyloric resistance. The American Journal of Physiology. 1985;**249**:G725-G732

[26] Keinke O, Schemann M, Ehrlein HJ. Mechanical factors regulating gastric-emptying of viscous nutrient meals in dogs. Quarterly Journal of Experimental Physiology and Cognate Medical Sciences. 1984;**69**:781-795

[27] Malbert CH, Ruckebusch Y. Duodenal bulb control of the flow-rate of digesta in the fasted and fed dog. Journal of Physiology (London). 1989;**409**:371-384

[28] Pallotta N, Cicala M, Frandina C, Corazziari E. Antro-pyloric contractile patterns and transpyloric flow after meal ingestion in humans. The American Journal of Gastroenterology. 1998;**93**:2513-2522

[29] Anvari M, Dent J, Jamieson GG. Mechanics of pulsatile transpyloric flow in the pig. Journal of Physiology (London). 1995;**488**:193-202

[30] Hausken T, Odegaard S, Matre K, Berstad A. Antroduodenal motility and movements of luminal contents studied by duplex sonography. Gastroenterology. 1992;**102**:1583-1590

[31] Malbert CH, Mathis C. Antropyloric modulation of transpyloric flow of liquids in pigs. Gastroenterology. 1994;**107**:37-46

[32] Horowitz M, Dent J, Fraser R, Sun W, Hebbard G. Role and integration of mechanisms controlling gastric emptying. Digestive Diseases and Sciences. 1994;**39**:7S-13S

[33] Houghton LA, Read NW, Heddle R, Maddern GJ, Downton J, Toouli J, et al. Motor activity of the gastric antrum, pylorus, and duodenum under fasted conditions and after a liquid meal. Gastroenterology. 1988;**94**:1276-1284

[34] Treacy PJ, Jamieson GG, Dent J. Pyloric motor function during emptying of a liquid meal from the stomach in the conscious pig. The Journal of Physiology. 1990;**422**:523-538

[35] Allescher HD, Daniel EE, Dent J, Fox JE, Kostolanska F. Extrinsic and intrinsic neural control of pyloric sphincter pressure in the dog. The Journal of Physiology. 1988;**401**:17-38

[36] Behar J, Biancani P, Zabinski MP. Characterization of feline gastroduodenal junction by neural and hormonal-stimulation. American Journal of Physiology. 1979;**236**:E45-E51

[37] Bertiger G, Reynolds JC, Ouyang A, Cohen S. Properties of the feline pyloric sphincter in vitro. Gastroenterology. 1987;**92**:1965-1972

[38] Brink BM, Schlegel JF, Code CF. The pressure profile of the gastroduodenal junctional zone in dogs. Gut. 1965;**6**:163-171

[39] Malbert CH, Mathis C, Laplace JP. Vagal control of pyloric resistance. The American Journal of Physiology. 1995;**269**:G558-G569

[40] Fraser R, Horowitz M, Dent J. Hyperglycaemia stimulates pyloric motility in normal subjects. Gut. 1991;**32**:475-478

[41] Heddle R, Fone D, Dent J, Horowitz M. Stimulation of pyloric motility by intraduodenal dextrose in normal subjects. Gut. 1988;**29**:1349-1357

[42] Tougas G, Anvari M, Dent J, Somers S, Richards D, Stevenson GW. Relation of pyloric motility to pyloric opening and closure in healthy subjects. Gut. 1992;**33**:466-471

[43] Heddle R, Dent J, Toouli J, Read NW. Topography and measurement of pyloric pressure waves and tone in humans. The American Journal of Physiology. 1988;**255**:G490-G497

[44] Avvari RK. Bio-mechanics of the distal stomach and duodenum: An insight into mechanisms of duodenogastric reflux and duodenal mixing. In: 48th Graduating Students Convocation. Kanpur: Indian Institute of Technology; 2015

[45] Thuneberg L, Peters S. Toward a concept of stretch-coupling in smooth muscle. I. Anatomy of intestinal segmentation and sleeve contractions. The Anatomical Record. 2001;**262**:110-124

[46] Wood JD. Enteric nervous control of motility in the upper gastrointestinal tract in defensive states. Digestive Diseases and Sciences. 1999;**44**:44S-52S

[47] Buhner S, Ehrlein HJ. Characteristics of postprandial duodenal motor patterns in dogs. Digestive Diseases and Sciences. 1989;**34**:1873-1881

[48] Dodds WJ, Stewart ET, Hodges D, Zboralske FF. Movement of the feline esophagus associated with respiration and peristalsis. An evaluation using tantalum markers. The Journal of Clinical Investigation. 1973;**52**:1-13

[49] Sugarbaker DJ, Rattan S, Goyal RK. Swallowing induces sequential activation of esophageal longitudinal smooth muscle. The American Journal of Physiology. 1984;**247**:G515-G519

[50] Pouderoux P, Lin S, Kahrilas PJ. Timing, propagation, coordination, and effect of esophageal shortening during peristalsis. Gastroenterology. 1997;**112**:1147-1154

[51] Edmundowicz SA, Clouse RE. Shortening of the esophagus in response to swallowing. The American Journal of Physiology. 1991;**260**:G512-G516

[52] Pal A, Brasseur JG. The mechanical advantage of local longitudinal shortening on peristaltic transport. Journal of Biomech Eng-T Asme. 2002;**124**:94-100

[53] Conklin JL. Nitric oxide: A mediator of esophageal motor function. The Journal of Laboratory and Clinical Medicine. 1998;**131**:10-20

[54] Li M, Brasseur JG. Non-steady peristaltic transport in finite-length tubes. Journal of Fluid Mechanics. 1993;**248**:129-151

[55] Inderjeeth AJ, Webberley KM, Muir J, Marshall BJ. The potential of computerised analysis of bowel sounds for diagnosis of gastrointestinal conditions: A systematic review. Systematic reviews. 2018;**7**:124

[56] Avvari RK. Effect of local longitudinal shortening on the transport of luminal contents through small intestine. Acta Mechanica Sinica. 2019;**35**

[57] Ewe K. Intestinal transport in constipation and diarrhoea. Pharmacology. 1988;**36**(Suppl 1):73-84

[58] Williams EK, Chang RB, Strochlic DE, Umans BD, Lowell BB, Liberles SD. Sensory neurons that detect stretch and nutrients in the digestive system. Cell. 2016;**166**:209-221

[59] Hur SJ, Decker EA, McClements DJ. Influence of initial emulsifier type on microstructural changes occurring in emulsified lipids during in vitro digestion. Food Chemistry. 2009;**114**:253-262

[60] Qin X, Wang X, Wang Y, Tang Z, Cui Q, Xi J, et al. MicroRNA-19a mediates the suppressive effect of laminar flow on cyclin D1 expression in human umbilical vein endothelial cells. Proceedings of the National Academy of Sciences of the United States of America. 2010;**107**:3240-3244

Section 2

Liver

Chapter 5

Serum Sodium Concentration in Patients with Portal Hypertension and Acute Gastrointestinal Bleeding Treated with Terlipressin: A Retrospective Observational Study

Xinmiao Zhou, Lichun Shao, Tingxue Song, Wenchun Bao, Xiaozhong Guo and Xingshun Qi

Abstract

This retrospective observational study aimed to investigate the risk of serum sodium concentration in patients treated with terlipressin and attempted to explore the factors associated with serum sodium concentration. We included 17 patients with portal hypertension treated with terlipressin (Group 1), 7 with portal hypertension treated with somatostatin/octreotide (Group 2), 20 with acute non-variceal gastrointestinal bleeding treated with somatostatin/octreotide (Group 3), and 19 with acute pancreatitis treated with somatostatin/octreotide (Group 4). In all groups, serum sodium concentration at baseline was not significantly different from the lowest value during the infusion of terlipressin, somatostatin, or octreotide (Group 1: 136.95 ± 4.68 versus 135.52 ± 4.79, $p = 0.426$; Group 2: 139.64 ± 3.86 versus 138.41 ± 5.34, $p = 0.813$; Group 3: 138.02 ± 4.08 versus 137.69 ± 3.11, $p = 0.630$; Group 4: 135.96 ± 6.87 versus 134.60 ± 3.40, $p = 0.098$). The rate of serum sodium concentration reduction in Group 1 (8/17) was not significantly different from Group 2 (3/7, $p = 1.000$), Group 3 (11/20, $p = 0.746$), or Group 4 (14/19, $p = 0.171$). Age, sex, baseline MELD and Child-Pugh scores, cDDD value and duration of terlipressin, blood transfusion, and diuretics and paracentesis during terlipressin were not significantly associated with serum sodium concentration reduction in Group 1. In conclusion, serum sodium concentration is often reduced in patients treated with terlipressin. However, the association of sodium concentration reduction with terlipressin should be clarified.

Keywords: hyponatremia, terlipressin, sodium, portal hypertension, gastrointestinal bleeding

1. Introduction

Terlipressin is a prodrug of vasopressin, which transforms into vasopressin by enzymatic cleavage of the glycyl residues [1, 2]. It has been approved as the choice of treatment for acute esophagogastric variceal bleeding (EGVB) [3–6]. Such a potent effect is mainly due to the activation of V1 receptors, which are dominantly located in the arterial smooth muscles of splanchnic circulation. The activation of V1 receptors causes the splanchnic vasoconstriction and thereby reduces the splanchnic blood flow and portal pressure [7]. In addition, terlipressin also activates the V2 receptors and increases the number of aquaporin-2 channels in the apical plasma membrane, thereby causing the water reabsorption in the renal collecting ducts [8]. This V2 receptor-mediated antidiuretic effect may result in dilutional hyponatremia. Mild to severe hyponatremia has been reported in a proportion of patients receiving terlipressin [9–12]. More notably, scattered case reports have also shown that patients with hyponatremia related to terlipressin develop the seizure [13–15].

Herein, this retrospective observational study aimed to investigate the risk of serum sodium concentration during terlipressin treatment and attempted to explore the factors associated with serum sodium concentration hyponatremia.

2. Materials and methods

Study protocol was reviewed and approved by the institutional review board of the General Hospital of Northern Theater Command (formally General Hospital of Shenyang Military Area).

2.1 Study population

All patients who were consecutively admitted to our department between February 2016 and November 2017 and were treated with terlipressin and/or somatostatin and/or octreotide by an attending physician (XQ) were considered as the study population.

Seventeen patients with portal hypertension who were diagnosed with acute gastrointestinal bleeding and were treated with terlipressin were considered as the experimental group (Group 1). Among them, 14 patients were diagnosed with liver cirrhosis due to hepatitis B virus alone (n = 5), hepatitis C virus plus alcohol abuse (n = 2), alcohol abuse alone (n = 2), autoimmune-related liver diseases alone (n = 2), drug-related liver diseases alone (n = 1), or unknown causes (n = 2); 4 patients had hepatocellular carcinoma; 15 patients underwent endoscopic examinations, of whom 6 and 9 had both esophageal and gastric varices and esophageal varices alone, respectively, but 2 patients refused; 9 patients received a combination of somatostatin (n = 6), octreotide (n = 1), and somatostatin plus octreotide (n = 2); 10 patients underwent endoscopic treatments, including esophageal variceal ligation alone (n = 6), esophageal sclerotherapy alone (n = 1), esophageal variceal ligation plus gastric tissue glue injection (n = 2), and esophageal sclerotherapy plus gastric tissue glue injection (n = 1).

Seven patients with portal hypertension who were diagnosed with acute gastrointestinal bleeding and were treated with somatostatin or octreotide but without terlipressin were considered as the first control group (Group 2). Among them, 6 patients were diagnosed with liver cirrhosis due to hepatitis B virus alone (n = 1), hepatitis B virus plus alcohol abuse (n = 2), alcohol abuse alone (n = 2), or unknown causes (n = 1); 2 patients had hepatocellular carcinoma; 6 patients underwent endoscopic examinations, of whom 3 and 3 had both esophageal and gastric varices and esophageal varices alone, respectively, but 1 patient was hemodynamically unstable and died before endoscopic examination; 4, 1, and 2 patients received somatostatin alone, octreotide alone, and somatostatin plus octreotide, respectively; and 5 patients underwent endoscopic treatments, including esophageal variceal ligation alone (n = 2), gastric tissue glue injection alone (n = 1), and esophageal variceal ligation plus gastric tissue glue injection (n = 2).

Twenty patients treated with somatostatin or octreotide for acute non-variceal gastrointestinal bleeding were considered as the second control group (Group 3). Among them, 15 patients underwent endoscopic examinations. The causes of bleeding were peptic ulcer (n = 9), acute gastric mucosal lesions (n = 1), gastric cancer (n = 1), Mallory-Weiss syndrome (n = 1), post-resection of colonic polyps (n = 1), colon cancer (n = 2), gastric occupation (n = 1), or unknown causes (n = 5).

Nineteen patients treated with somatostatin or octreotide for acute pancreatitis were considered as the third control group (Group 4).

2.2 Terlipressin

Terlipressin (Ferring Pharmaceuticals, Kiel, Germany) was given by continuous intravenous infusion 1 mg every 6 hours in 16 patients and intravenous bolus 1 mg followed by continuous intravenous infusion 1 mg every 6 hours in 1 patient. Terlipressin can be maintained for a maximum of 5 days [16]. Terlipressin was discontinued till bleeding ceased for 72 hours (no hematemesis and melena) or patients received successful endoscopic treatments.

2.3 Somatostatin/octreotide

Somatostatin was given by continuous intravenous infusion 3 mg every 12 hours. Octreotide was given by continuous intravenous infusion 0.3 mg every 12 hours or subcutaneous injection 0.1 mg every 8 hours depending upon the severity of diseases. Somatostatin and octreotide can be used for 5 days or even longer [3]. As for patients with acute gastrointestinal bleeding, somatostatin or octreotide was discontinued till bleeding ceased for 72 hours (no hematemesis and melena) or patients received successful endoscopic treatments. As for patients with acute pancreatitis, somatostatin/octreotide was discontinued till abdominal symptoms disappeared, serum amylase and lipase levels returned to the normal range or was close to the normal range, inflammation parameters levels returned to the normal range, and peri-pancreatic exudation disappeared or remarkably reduced.

2.4 Data collection

Baseline data refer to the data recorded before terlipressin, somatostatin, or octreotide was initiated. They included demographic information; etiology of liver cirrhosis; major clinical presentations, such as hepatic encephalopathy, acute upper gastrointestinal bleeding, and ascites; major laboratory tests, such as white blood cell, hemoglobin, platelet count, total bilirubin, albumin, alanine aminotransferase, aspartate aminotransferase, blood urea nitrogen, serum creatinine, potassium, serum sodium, prothrombin time, activated partial thromboplastin time, international normalized ratio, D-Dimer, Model for End-Stage Liver Disease (MELD) and Child-Pugh scores, blood transfusion, amount of red blood cell transfused, diuretics and paracentesis, and duration of terlipressin, somatostatin, and octreotide.

We screened the hepatic and renal function, blood cell counts, and serum electrolytes during hospitalization depending upon the patients' profiles. The lowest serum sodium concentration was collected when terlipressin, somatostatin, or octreotide was being given.

We also recorded the first re-examination value during the infusion of terlipressin and the value after stopping the infusion of terlipressin.

2.5 Outcomes

The primary end point of the study was to investigate the changes of serum sodium concentration during the administration of terlipressin and/or somatostatin and/or octreotide. The changes of serum sodium concentration were compared (i.e., the baseline value versus the lowest value or the value after stopping the pharmacological treatment). The rate of serum sodium concentration reduction among groups was assessed.

In the Group 1, we evaluated the difference between the baseline and lowest value of serum sodium during the treatment and classified as sodium decreased and sodium stable or increased. The secondary end point was to assess the factors associated with serum sodium concentration reduction in patients treated with terlipressin for portal hypertension.

2.6 Statistical analysis

Continuous variables were presented as mean ± standard deviations and medians with ranges, and categorical variables as frequency (%). Comparison of continuous variables between groups was performed by using Mann-Whitney U-test and paired comparison rank sum test, and that of categorical variables by using Chi-square or Fisher's exact test. The statistical analyses were performed by using SPSS version 24.0 (SPSS Inc., Chicago, IL, USA) and GraphPad Prism version 6.0 (7825 Fay Avenue, Suite 230, La Jolla, CA 92037, USA). $p < 0.05$ for the difference was statistically significant.

3. Results

3.1 Patient characteristics

Overall, 17, 7, 20, and 19 patients were included in Group 1, 2, 3, and 4, respectively (**Figure 1**). Characteristics of patients are shown in **Table 1**.

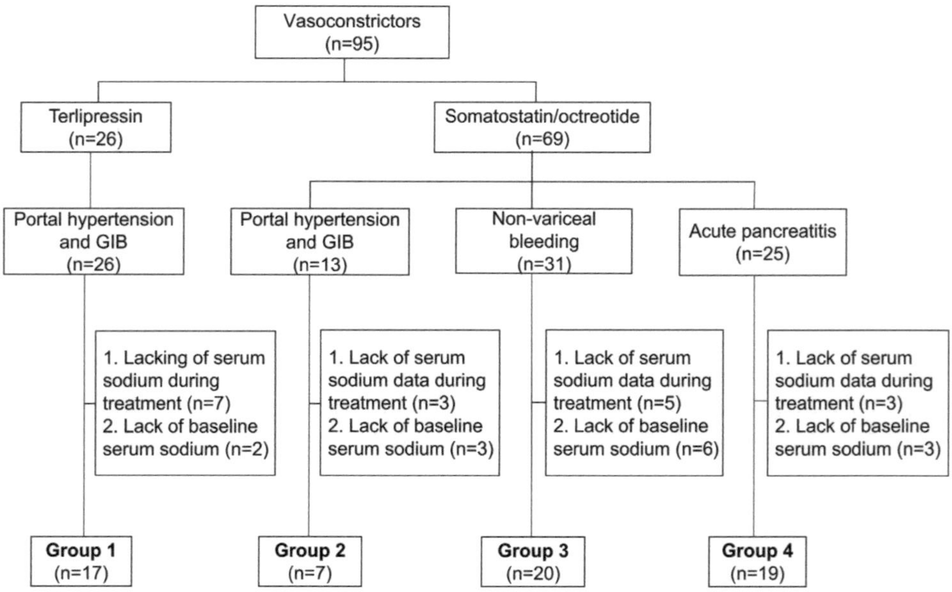

Figure 1.
Flow chart of patient enrollment. Abbreviations: GIB, gastrointestinal bleeding.

DOI: http://dx.doi.org/10.5772/intechopen.89981

Variables	Group 1			Group 2			Group 3			Group 4		
	No. pts	Mean ± SD or n (%)	Median (range)	No. pts	Mean ± SD or n (%)	Median (range)	No. pts	Mean ± SD or n (%)	Median (range)	No. pts	Mean ± SD or n (%)	Median (range)
Age (years)	17	58.06 ± 11.04	57 (34–75)	7	54.57 ± 9.54	52 (42–71)	20	59.10 ± 20.24	57 (20–93)	19	53.89 ± 20.53	49 (28–84)
Sex—male, n (%)	17	9 (52.9%)	—	7	6 (85.7%)	—	20	15 (75%)	—	19	14 (73.7%)	—
Clinical presentations												
Hepatic encephalopathy, n (%)	17	1 (5.9%)	—	7	0 (0)	—	20	—	—	19	—	—
Upper gastrointestinal bleeding, n (%)	17	17 (100%)	—	7	7 (100%)	—	20	17 (85%)	—	19	—	—
Ascites, n (%)	17	12 (70.6%)	—	7	1 (14.3%)	—	20	—	—	19	—	—
Laboratory tests												
White blood cell (10^9/L)	17	6.08 ± 3.92	4.9 (1.5–18.5)	7	5.4 ± 2.29	4.3 (2.2–8.4)	20	9.66 ± 5.54	8.65 (4.3–28.9)	19	9.42 ± 4.11	8.7 (2.1–16.5)
Hemoglobin (g/L)	17	71.65 ± 21.14	72 (37–124)	7	85.00 ± 17.25	79 (70–119)	20	93.95 ± 29.40	91.5 (48–136)	19	138.21 ± 31.10	135 (83–205)
Platelet count (10^9/L)	17	117.65 ± 93.00	82 (29–387)	7	115.14 ± 43.97	118 (59–174)	20	305.20 ± 274.58	238 (98–1287)	19	223.89 ± 87.69	221 (41–434)
Total bilirubin (umol/L)	17	28.25 ± 24.39	17.2 (8.1–92.3)	7	24.19 ± 14.83	16.6 (8.3–49.1)	20	12.29 ± 8.71	9.15 (3.5–33.7)	19	50.87 ± 59.56	19.6 (10–213.3)
Albumin (g/L)	17	29.09 ± 5.19	29.8 (18.7–39.1)	7	27.67 ± 5.21	25.6 (22–36.3)	20	34.24 ± 4.70	33.65 (24.8–41.5)	18	37 ± 6.46	37.4 (25.8–49.3)
Alanine aminotransferase (U/L)	17	22.41 ± 17.96	14.71 (10.13–77.1)	7	19.85 ± 7.34	22.02 (10.57–28.38)	20	17.93 ± 14.75	15.05 (4.57–65)	19	91.44 ± 97.24	49.12 (5.06–311.04)
Aspartate aminotransferase (U/L)	17	32.13 ± 18.14	25.05 (17.17–89.1)	7	33.00 ± 16.81	29.61 (17.88–65.85)	19	21.64 ± 12.29	15.5 (10.3–58)	19	83.15 ± 100.04	37.22 (13.79–369.2)
Blood urea nitrogen (mmol/L)	17	10.31 ± 5.54	9.39 (4.11–25.97)	7	7.44 ± 2.05	8.85 (3.86–9.05)	20	10.49 ± 6.14	8.79 (3.03–23.27)	19	5.72 ± 2.36	5.29 (2.09–11.21)
Serum creatinine (umol/L)	17	67.71 ± 21.71	62.78 (31.85–117.38)	7	107.67 ± 93.20	67.3 (52.65–314)	20	77.00 ± 27.05	67.05 (42–147)	19	66.02 ± 27.36	73.9 (18.32–129.9)
Potassium (mmol/L)	17	4.09 ± 0.69	3.84 (3.1–6.03)	7	4.07 ± 0.50	4.16 (3.33–4.64)	20	4.06 ± 0.48	3.99 (3.25–4.99)	19	4.01 ± 0.65	4.04 (2.86–5.84)
Sodium (mmol/L)	17	136.95 ± 4.68	137.4 (126.3–142.9)	7	139.64 ± 3.86	141.2 (132–142.7)	20	138.02 ± 4.08	138.35 (126.6–144)	19	135.96 ± 6.86	137.4 (115.1–142.6)
Prothrombin time (seconds)	17	17.13 ± 2.30	16.5 (15–23.9)	7	16.76 ± 2.23	17 (14.7–20.8)	19	14.90 ± 2.93	13.8 (12.9–24.9)	18	14.46 ± 3.26	13.3 (12–23.4)

Variables	Group 1			Group 2			Group 3			Group 4		
	No. pts	Mean ± SD or n (%)	Median (range)	No. pts	Mean ± SD or n (%)	Median (range)	No. pts	Mean ± SD or n (%)	Median (range)	No. pts	Mean ± SD or n (%)	Median (range)
Activated partial thromboplastin time (seconds)	17	38.21 ± 5.11	37.4 (29–47.8)	7	39.07 ± 4.25	40.2 (34.6–44.5)	19	33.56 ± 5.67	33.1 (25.6–47.9)	18	35.68 ± 6.20	34.6 (29.2–50.1)
International normalized ratio	17	1.45 ± 0.30	1.34 (1.16–2.08)	7	1.38 ± 0.25	1.39 (1.14–1.83)	19	1.17 ± 0.31	1.05 (0.95–2.24)	18	1.32 ± 0.34	1 (0.88–2.08)
D-Dimer (mg/L)	17	2.09 ± 2.23	1.09 (0.15–7.39)	7	1.85 ± 2.29	1.02 (0.38–6.86)	19	2.90 ± 10.40	0.33 (0.1–45.81)	17	2.42 ± 2.70	1.51 (0.24–9.38)
Model for end-stage liver disease score	17	8.23 ± 4.68	8.58 (0.9–16.84)	7	10.48 ± 5.60	11.05 (3.1–19.72)	—	—	—	—	—	—
Child-Pugh score	17	7.76 ± 1.92	7 (5–12)	7	7.14 ± 1.77	7 (5–10)	—	—	—	—	—	—
Duration of terlipressin (days)	17	3.15 ± 1.18	3 (1.25–5)	—	—	—	—	—	—	—	—	—
Duration of somatostatin or octreotide (days)	—	—	—	7	6.79 ± 4.58	6.5 (1.5–14.5)	20	3.88 ± 2.54	3 (0.25–12)	19	10.36 ± 5.14	10 (2–20)
Blood transfusion, n (%)	17	11 (64.7%)	—	7	4 (57.1%)	—	20	9 (45.0%)	—	—	—	—
Amount of red blood cell transfused (U)	11	5.06 ± 1.77	5 (2–8)	4	3.38 ± 1.38	3.25 (2–5)	9	2.39 ± 1.43	2 (1–5.5)	—	—	—

Group 1, terlipressin in portal hypertension;
Group 2, somatostatin or octreotide in portal hypertension;
Group 3, somatostatin or octreotide in non-variceal gastrointestinal bleeding;
Group 4, somatostatin or octreotide in acute pancreatitis.

Table 1.
Characteristics of patients.

3.2 Change in serum sodium concentration

Group 1. Serum sodium concentration before the infusion of terlipressin was not significantly different from the lowest value during the infusion of terlipressin (136.95 ± 4.68 versus 135.52 ± 4.79, p = 0.426) (**Figure 2A**), the first re-examination value during the infusion of terlipressin (136.24 ± 4.97, p = 0.989) (**Figure 2B**), or the value after stopping the infusion of terlipressin (136.29 ± 2.86, p = 0.926) (**Figure 2C**).

Group 2. Serum sodium concentration before the infusion of somatostatin or octreotide was not significantly different from the lowest value during the infusion of somatostatin or octreotide (139.64 ± 3.86 versus 138.41 ± 5.34, p = 0.813) (**Figure 2D**).

Group 3. Serum sodium concentration before the infusion of somatostatin or octreotide was not significantly different from the lowest value during the infusion of somatostatin or octreotide (138.02 ± 4.08 versus 137.69 ± 3.11, p = 0.630) (**Figure 2E**).

Group 4. Serum sodium concentration before the infusion of somatostatin or octreotide was not significantly different from the lowest value during the infusion of somatostatin or octreotide (135.96 ± 6.87 versus 134.60 ± 3.40, p = 0.098) (**Figure 2F**).

3.3 Percentage of patients who developed serum sodium concentration reduction among groups

The percentage of patients who developed serum sodium concentration reduction in Group 1 (8/17, 47.1%) was not significantly different from Group 2 (3/7,

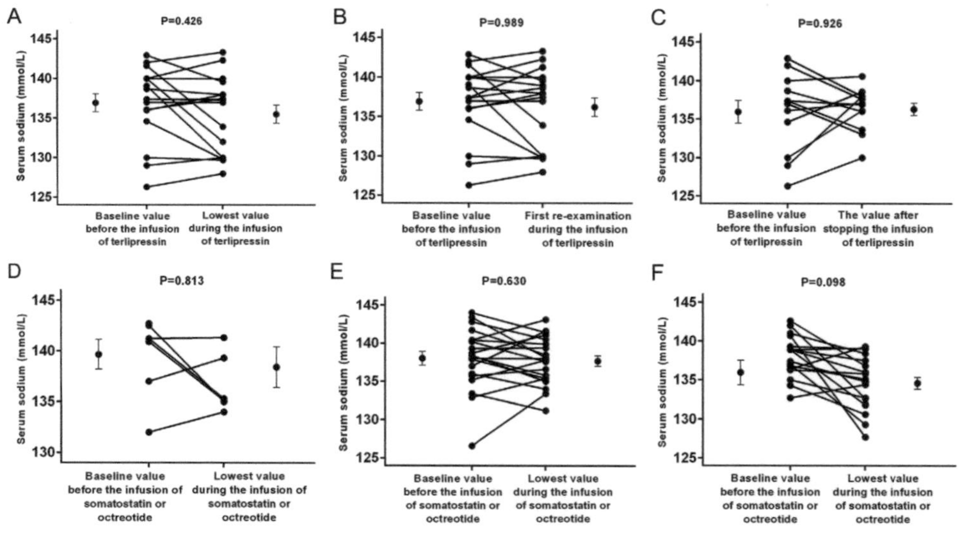

Figure 2.
Change in serum sodium concentration. (A) Serum sodium concentration before the infusion of terlipressin versus the lowest value during the infusion of terlipressin in Group 1. (B) Serum sodium concentration before the infusion of terlipressin versus the first re-examination value during the infusion of terlipressin in Group 1. (C) Serum sodium concentration before the infusion of terlipressin versus the value after stopping the infusion of terlipressin in Group 1. (D) Serum sodium concentration before the infusion of somatostatin or octreotide versus the lowest value during the infusion of somatostatin or octreotide in Group 2. (E) Serum sodium concentration before the infusion of somatostatin or octreotide versus the lowest value during the infusion of somatostatin or octreotide in Group 3. (F) Serum sodium concentration before the infusion of somatostatin or octreotide versus the lowest value during the infusion of somatostatin or octreotide in Group 4.

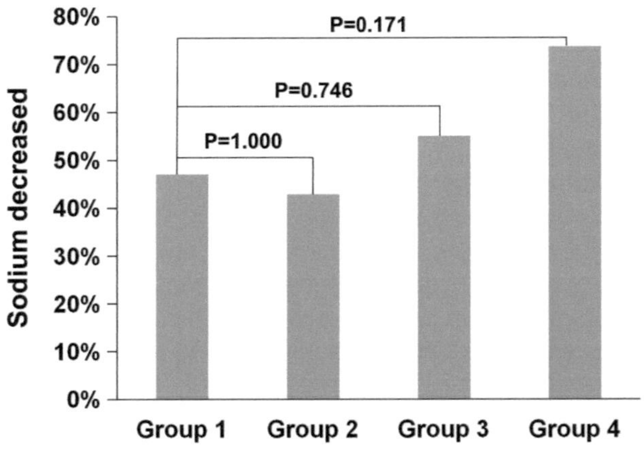

Figure 3.
Percentage of patients who developed serum sodium concentration reduction among groups.

42.9%, p = 1.000), Group 3 (11/20, 55%, p = 0.746), or Group 4 (14/19, 73.7%, p = 0.171) (**Figure 3**).

3.4 Factors associated with serum sodium concentration reduction in Group 1

Age, sex, baseline MELD and Child-Pugh scores, cDDD value and duration of terlipressin, blood transfusion, and diuretics and paracentesis during terlipressin were not significantly associated with serum sodium concentration reduction (**Table 2**).

Variables	Sodium decreased			Sodium stable or increased			P value
	No. pts	Mean ± SD or n (%)	Median (range)	No. pts	Mean ± SD or n (%)	Median (range)	
Age (years)	8	57.38 ± 10.18	59 (44–73)	9	58.67 ± 12.34	57 (34–75)	0.819
Sex—male, n (%)	8	3 (37.5%)	—	9	6 (66.7%)	—	0.347
Clinical presentations							
Hepatic encephalopathy, n (%)	8	0	—	9	1 (11.1%)	—	1.000
Upper gastrointestinal bleeding, n (%)	8	8 (100%)	—	9	9 (100%)	—	—
Ascites, n (%)	8	5 (62.5%)	—	9	7 (77.8%)	—	0.620
Laboratory tests							
White blood cell (10^9/L)	8	5.38 ± 2.23	4.7 (2.9–8.5)	9	6.72 ± 5.04	5 (1.5–18.5)	0.773
Hemoglobin (g/L)	8	74.5 ± 7.45	74 (64–85)	9	69.11 ± 28.80	60 (37–124)	0.360
Platelet count (10^9/L)	8	113.13 ± 63.75	92.5 (40–237)	9	121.67 ± 117.06	76 (29–387)	0.441
Total bilirubin (umol/L)	8	30.91 ± 25.64	25.5 (12.8–92.3)	9	25.87 ± 24.52	13.4 (8.1–79.9)	0.248

DOI: http://dx.doi.org/10.5772/intechopen.89981

Variables	Sodium decreased			Sodium stable or increased			P value
	No. pts	Mean ± SD or n (%)	Median (range)	No. pts	Mean ± SD or n (%)	Median (range)	
Albumin (g/L)	8	29.06 ± 5.92	29.4 (18.7–39.1)	9	29.11 ± 4.81	29.8 (19–35.3)	0.847
Alanine aminotransferase (U/L)	8	23.35 ± 22.08	16.67 (10.13–77.1)	9	21.58 ± 14.73	14.69 (11.89–56.9)	0.923
Aspartate aminotransferase (U/L)	8	30.91 ± 12.85	25.51 (17.17–52.5)	9	33.21 ± 22.60	24.64 (17.22–89.1)	0.773
Blood urea nitrogen (mmol/L)	8	11.1 ± 6.54	9.6 (4.56–25.97)	9	9.60 ± 4.77	9.24 (4.11–18.83)	0.700
Serum creatinine (umol/L)	8	70.38 ± 30.66	68.53 (31.85–117.38)	9	65.33 ± 10.31	62.78 (50–78.35)	0.847
Potassium (mmol/L)	8	4.22 ± 0.76	4.01 (3.72–6.03)	9	3.98 ± 0.64	3.8 (3.1–5.21)	0.290
Sodium (mmol/L)	8	138.04 ± 4.12	138.9 (130–142.9)	9	135.98 ± 5.17	137 (126.3–142)	0.359
Prothrombin time (seconds)	8	16.95 ± 2.02	16.25 (15–20.4)	9	17.29 ± 2.63	16.8 (15.1–23.9)	0.629
Activated partial thromboplastin time (seconds)	8	39.06 ± 6.12	39.7 (30.6–47.8)	9	37.44 ± 4.26	37.3 (29–44.8)	0.501
D-Dimer (mg/L)	8	2.14 ± 2.13	1.3 (0.37–6.45)	9	2.05 ± 2.44	1.07 (0.15–7.39)	0.630
Ammonia (umol/L)	7	49.57 ± 19.44	53 (9–71)	8	50 ± 18.75	56.5 (19–72)	0.772
Model for End-Stage Liver Disease score	8	8.61 ± 5.69	9.49 (0.9–16.84)	9	7.87 ± 3.88	7.56 (1.94–15.06)	0.847
Child-Pugh score	8	7.75 ± 2.12	7 (6–12)	9	7.78 ± 1.86	8 (5–11)	0.807
cDDD value of terlipressin	8	1.15 ± 0.46	1.13 (0.5–1.67)	9	1.01 ± 0.41	1 (0.42–1.67)	0.530
Duration of terlipressin (days)	8	3.25 ± 1.22	3.13 (1.5–5)	9	3.03 ± 1.22	3 (1.25–5)	0.699
Blood transfusion, n (%)	8	4 (50%)	—	9	7 (77.8%)	—	0.335
Amount of red blood cell transfused (U)	4	4.5 ± 1.73	5 (2–6)	7	5.39 ± 1.84	5.2 (2–8)	0.331
Diuretics during terlipressin, n (%)	8	1 (12.5%)	—	9	1 (11.1%)	—	1.000
Paracentesis during terlipressin, n (%)	8	0	—	9	0	—	—

Table 2.
Factors associated with serum sodium concentration reduction in patients treated with terlipressin.

4. Discussion

In the present study, approximately half of our patients receiving terlipressin developed serum sodium concentration reduction after short-term treatment with terlipressin (3.15 ± 1.18 days). The incidence of hyponatremia or serum sodium concentration reduction was often heterogeneous among studies due to the characteristics of patients enrolled; definitions of hyponatremia or serum sodium concentration reduction; and indications, approaches, durations, and dosages of terlipressin. In randomized controlled trials regarding terlipressin for the treatment of EGVB, the incidence of hyponatremia, which was defined as serum sodium <130 mmol/L, was 0–6% [17–20]. Sola et al. [10] found that the incidence of serum sodium decreased >10 mmol/L from the baseline was 36% (21/58) in patients with EGVB treated by terlipressin for 5 days. Yim et al. [12] found that the incidence of serum sodium decreased >10 mmol/L from the baseline was 26.5% (40/151) in patients with EGVB treated by terlipressin for 5 days. Kang et al. [11] also reported that the incidence of serum sodium decreased >5 mmol/L from the baseline was 35.4% (45/127) during or after terlipressin treatment in patients with EGVB and hepatorenal syndrome (HRS).

Theoretically, terlipressin can induce the reduction of serum sodium concentration, because it activates the V2 receptors, thereby increasing the number of aquaporin-2 water channels in the apical plasma membrane and causing the water reabsorption in the renal collecting ducts [8]. However, there is little effect of terlipressin on V2 receptors, which is equal to only 3% of antidiuretic effect of vasopressin [13]. Indeed, the present study did not find any severe hyponatremia in our patients receiving terlipressin. Additionally, serum sodium concentration change (i.e., the baseline value versus the lowest value or the first re-examination value) was not statistically significant in all patients receiving terlipressin.

Somatostatin and its analogues cause the splanchnic vasoconstriction mainly by inhibiting the production and release of vasodilators, such as glucagon and vasoactive intestinal peptide, to reduce the portal pressure [6, 21]. They do not cause the change of serum sodium concentration. Thus, in order to further explore the effect of terlipressin on serum sodium concentration, the present study also compared the risk of serum sodium concentration reduction between patients receiving terlipressin and those receiving somatostatin or octreotide. We found that serum sodium concentration change in patients receiving terlipressin was not different from those receiving somatostatin or octreotide. These findings also suggested little effect of terlipressin on serum sodium concentration.

Several previous studies reported the risk factors for hyponatremia due to terlipressin. In 2010, Sola et al. [10] found that high baseline serum sodium level and low MELD score were independent risk factors for decreased serum sodium level. In 2013, Kang et al. [11] found that high baseline serum sodium level was an independent risk factor for hyponatremia. In 2015, Yim et al. [12] found that younger age, lower Child-Pugh score, higher baseline serum sodium, and long-term use of terlipressin (>5 days) were independent risk factors for hyponatremia and that lower body mass index and Child-Pugh score and higher baseline serum sodium were independent risk factors for rapid and severe hyponatremia. In 2017, Kim et al. [9] found that hepatitis B, diabetes mellitus, baseline serum sodium and creatinine levels, and shock at admission were independent risk factors for hyponatremia. Taken together, higher baseline serum sodium level and better liver function (low MELD or Child-Pugh score) are risk factors for hyponatremia during the treatment with terlipressin. In patients with more severe liver dysfunction, the portal pressure might be higher and the release of endogenous vasopressin was increased, thereby occupying the V2 vasopressin receptor. Thus, the antidiuretic effect of terlipressin is compromised. We attempted to explore the baseline factors associated with serum sodium concentration reduction during terlipressin. Unfortunately, the duration of terlipressin, cDDD value of terlipressin, blood transfusion, amount of blood transfusion, and diuretics and paracentesis during terlipressin were not significantly associated with serum sodium concentration reduction. Certainly, this analysis should be performed again in a larger number of patients.

The duration, dosage, and route of terlipressin may be also associated with the risk of hyponatremia related to terlipressin. Bruha et al. [22] conducted a multicenter randomized double-blind study to compare the efficacy and safety of 10-day versus 5-day terlipressin for the treatment of EGVB, and found that prolonged terlipressin treatment was the only risk factor of hyponatremia. Chang et al. [23] conducted a randomized controlled study to compare the efficacy and safety of high-dose versus low-dose terlipressin for the treatment of EGVB. They did not find any patient with hyponatremia in both groups. Cavallin et al. [24] conducted a randomized controlled study to compare continuous intravenous infusion versus intravenous bolus terlipressin for type 1 HRS. Similarly, they found that no patient developed hyponatremia in both groups. By comparison, in the present study, we prescribed a relatively short duration of terlipressin and minimized the dosage of terlipressin.

There are several limitations in the present study. First, the patient characteristics were heterogeneous in the Group 1. Second, this was a single-center retrospective cohort study, and the sample size was small. Third, a combination of somatostatin and/or octreotide was also given in some of our patients. Fourth, the time point when we re-checked the serum sodium concentration was defined according to the patients' conditions and disease course. Thus, it was not uniform among patients.

In conclusion, serum sodium concentration reduction can be observed in patients with portal hypertension during terlipressin treatment. However, this phenomenon might not be closely associated with the use of terlipressin. The present study failed to identify any factors associated with serum sodium concentration reduction. Future studies with a larger number of patients should be performed to validate our findings.

Acknowledgements

This work was partially presented as a poster presentation at the 18th Congress of Gastroenterology China that was held in Dalian, China, on September 2018.

Conflict of interest

None.

Funding

None.

Author contributions

Xinmiao Zhou wrote the protocol, collected the data, performed the statistical analysis, interpreted the data, and drafted the manuscript. Tingxue Song wrote the protocol, collected the data, and performed the statistical analysis. Wenchun Bao wrote the protocol, collected the data, and checked the data. Lichun Shao and Xiaozhong Guo checked the data and gave critical comments Xingshun Qi conceived the work, wrote the protocol, performed the statistical analysis, interpreted the data, and revised the manuscript.

Author details

Xinmiao Zhou[1,2,3], Lichun Shao[3], Tingxue Song[3], Wenchun Bao[1], Xiaozhong Guo[1] and Xingshun Qi[1*]

1 Department of Gastroenterology, General Hospital of Northern Theater Command (formally General Hospital of Shenyang Military Area), Shenyang, P.R. China

2 Postgraduate College, Jinzhou Medical University, Jinzhou, P.R. China

3 Department of Gastroenterology, No. 463 Hospital of Chinese PLA, Shenyang, P.R. China

*Address all correspondence to: xingshunqi@126.com

References

[1] Hansen EF, Strandberg C, Hojgaard L, et al. Splanchnic haemodynamics after intravenous terlipressin in anaesthetised healthy pigs. Journal of Hepatology. 1999;**30**(3): 503-510

[2] Sarin SK, Sharma P. Terlipressin: An asset for hepatologists! Hepatology. 2011;**54**(2):724-728

[3] Garcia-Tsao G, Sanyal AJ, Grace ND, et al. Prevention and management of gastroesophageal varices and variceal hemorrhage in cirrhosis. Hepatology. 2007;**46**(3):922-938

[4] de Franchis R. Expanding consensus in portal hypertension: Report of the Baveno VI consensus workshop: Stratifying risk and individualizing care for portal hypertension. Journal of Hepatology. 2015;**63**(3): 743-752

[5] de Franchis R. Revising consensus in portal hypertension: Report of the Baveno V consensus workshop on methodology of diagnosis and therapy in portal hypertension. Journal of Hepatology. 2010;**53**(4): 762-768

[6] D'Amico G, Pagliaro L, Bosch J. Pharmacological treatment of portal hypertension: An evidence-based approach. Seminars in Liver Disease. 1999;**19**(4):475-505

[7] Moller S, Hansen EF, Becker U, et al. Central and systemic haemodynamic effects of terlipressin in portal hypertensive patients. Liver. 2000; **20**(1):51-59

[8] Krag A, Bendtsen F, Pedersen EB, et al. Effects of terlipressin on the aquaretic system: Evidence of antidiuretic effects. American Journal of Physiology Renal Physiology. 2008; **295**(5):F1295-F1300

[9] Kim SE, Jung DM, Park JW, et al. Baseline renal function predicts hyponatremia in liver cirrhosis patients treated with terlipressin for variceal bleeding. Gastroenterology Research and Practice. 2017;**2017**:7610374

[10] Sola E, Lens S, Guevara M, et al. Hyponatremia in patients treated with terlipressin for severe gastrointestinal bleeding due to portal hypertension. Hepatology. 2010;**52**(5):1783-1790

[11] Kang YJ, Bae EJ, Hwang K, et al. Initial serum sodium concentration determines the decrease in sodium level after terlipressin administration in patients with liver cirrhosis. Springerplus. 2013;**2**:519

[12] Yim SY, Seo YS, Jung CH, et al. Risk factors for developing hyponatremia during terlipressin treatment: A retrospective analyses in variceal bleeding. Journal of Clinical Gastroenterology. 2015;**49**(7):607-612

[13] Dunwoodie E, Jowett S. Terlipressin causing a hyponatraemic seizure. Scandinavian Journal of Gastroenterology. 2007;**42**(5):665

[14] Hyun JJ, Seo YS, Lee KG, et al. Terlipressin-induced hyponatremic seizure. Scandinavian Journal of Gastroenterology. 2010;**45**(4):501-504

[15] Zaki SA. Terlipressin-induced hyponatremic seizure in a child. Indian Journal of Pharmacology. 2013;**45**(4): 403-404

[16] Garcia-Tsao G, Bosch J. Management of varices and variceal hemorrhage in cirrhosis. The New England Journal of Medicine. 2010; **362**(9):823-832

[17] Abid S, Jafri W, Hamid S, et al. Terlipressin vs. octreotide in bleeding esophageal varices as an adjuvant

therapy with endoscopic band ligation: A randomized double-blind placebo-controlled trial. The American Journal of Gastroenterology. 2009;**104**(3):617-623

[18] Escorsell A, Ruiz del Arbol L, Planas R, et al. Multicenter randomized controlled trial of terlipressin versus sclerotherapy in the treatment of acute variceal bleeding: The TEST study. Hepatology. 2000;**32**(3):471-476

[19] Feu F, Ruiz del Arbol L, Banares R, et al. Double-blind randomized controlled trial comparing terlipressin and somatostatin for acute variceal hemorrhage. Variceal Bleeding Study Group. Gastroenterology. 1996;**111**(5): 1291-1299

[20] Lo GH, Chen WC, Wang HM, et al. Low-dose terlipressin plus banding ligation versus low-dose terlipressin alone in the prevention of very early rebleeding of oesophageal varices. Gut. 2009;**58**(9):1275-1280

[21] Bhutta AQ, Garcia-Tsao G. The role of medical therapy for variceal bleeding. Gastrointestinal Endoscopy Clinics of North America. 2015;**25**(3):479-490

[22] Bruha R, Marecek Z, Prochazka V, et al. Double-blind randomized multicenter study comparing the efficacy and safety of 10-day to 5-day terlipressin treatment of bleeding esophageal varices. Hepato-Gastroenterology. 2009;**56**(90):390-394

[23] Chang TT, Lee FY, Tsai YT, et al. A randomized controlled study of low-dose and high-dose terlipressin in the control of acute oesophageal variceal haemorrhage. Journal of Gastroenterology and Hepatology. 1991; **6**(5):481-484

[24] Cavallin M, Piano S, Romano A, et al. Terlipressin given by continuous intravenous infusion versus intravenous boluses in the treatment of hepatorenal syndrome: A randomized controlled study. Hepatology. 2016;**63**(3):983-992

Section 3

Biliary System

Chapter 6

Prologue: Biliary System - History and Background

Sam Koruth and Sooraj Sankar

1. Introduction

Cholecystectomy is one of the most common surgeries performed all around the world; over 600,000 people in the US undergo cholecystectomies each year. It is the treatment of choice for inflammation of the gallbladder (cholecystitis), pain and inflammation related to gall stones (calculus cholecystitis) and pancreatitis caused by gall stones.

Carl Johann August Langenbuch, a 27-year-old director of the Lazarus Hospital in Berlin, first practiced cholecystectomy on a cadaver, and then in the year 1882, he performed a cholecystectomy on a man who had suffered from gallstones for 16 years and cured his painful condition overnight. He was initially frustrated and disturbed that his patients continued to suffer after minor procedures to drain or clean the gallbladder, and then he became determined to give these patients a cure rather than temporary relief, and thus the first open cholecystectomy captured the history books.

By 1897, over 100 cholecystectomies had been performed, and it turned out that the removal of the gallbladder not only would not take life but could in fact provide a pain-free future. Then in 1985, the modern era of cholecystectomies began when the surgeon Erich Mühe of Böblingen, Germany, did the first endoscopic cholecystectomy. Thereafter the pioneers in France and the US surgeons attached a CCD video camera to a laparoscope allowing the surgical team to view the operative field and perform with laparoscopic instruments. A French gynecologic surgeon performed a laparoscopic gallbladder removal in 1987. Soon after that in just 2 years, demand for the laparoscopic approach transformed surgical practice in the US and other countries and subsequently recognized laparoscopic cholecystectomies as the gold standard treatment for gallstone disease. The benefits of the laparoscopic approach were ultimately codified in the new National Institutes of Health (NIH) guidelines in 1992, and they stated that it provided a safe and effective treatment for most patients with symptomatic gallstones.

To date, it is documented that more than 80% of the cholecystectomies are done via laparoscopic approach. The advantages of laparoscopic over open surgeries are quite clear. These advantages include shorter length of hospital stay, very less operative pain, avoiding a big scar over the abdomen, earlier return of bowel function, improved cosmesis, earlier return to normal activities and overall decreased cost. The rates of cholecystectomies have increased subsequently with the introduction of laparoscopic procedures accompanied by evidence of lower clinical thresholds for operative therapy of gallstone diseases.

2. Tips for a safe cholecystectomy

I have personally penned down certain points in my personal experience which can be used as a guide or may be even as a checklist before the young talented surgeons place their hands on cholecystectomies:

1. Selection of initial cases—female thin built patients with short history of biliary colics and especially no history of cholecystitis as there would be adhesions and would be a task to dissect during the initial days.

2. Informed consent including chances of conversion and high risk of various injuries to bile duct or other nearby structures.

3. Proper cleaning and sterilization of instruments.

4. Good quality equipment and instruments.

5. A good first assistant and a qualified and trained surgeon.

6. Formal training in laparoscopic surgeries to have a basic knowledge about the instruments and the technique.

7. 30° telescope.

8. Open technique of first port.

9. Urine to be evacuated just before the surgery.

10. Fundus should be retracted towards the right shoulder.

11. Vascular anatomy and biliary tract anatomies are different and vary from person to person.

12. Consider cystic lymph node of Lund as a guide for the cystic duct.

13. Hydrodissection and suction cannula can be a good instrument for blunt dissection.

14. It is safer to leave a few mm of cystic duct than to shave it off near to the common bile duct.

15. Double clips are always safer on the patient side of the structures.

16. Cystic ducts can be wider, longer, tortuous, double or even very short.

17. Fundus-first techniques can be adopted for difficult cases.

18. Bleeding seen on the screen will usually be less as they are magnified versions.

19. All bleedings will stop with pressure except the physiological menstrual bleed. So in case if there is bleeding, avoid panic, give pressure with gauze piece and control the bleed.

20. Partial cholecystectomies are an option for difficult cases.

21. Do not hesitate to open the abdomen in case of bleeding or difficult anatomy.

22. All stumps should be carefully examined.

23. Bile spillage and stone spillage should be sucked out or removed.

24. Conversions are not failures, and surgeons should not have an ego to finish all cases via a laparoscopic approach.

25. Whatever taken out of the body including all gallbladders should be sent for histopathology.

3. Gallstone pancreatitis

Acute pancreatitis is now the most common reason for hospital admission among all gastrointestinal disorders [1]. Population-based studies indicate that the incidence of acute pancreatitis is rising from 14.8 in 100,000 (1990–1994) to 31.2 in 100,000 (2010–2013) among British males [2]. The most common (about 30–50%) preventable cause of pancreatitis in the United Kingdom is gallstones [3]. Recurrent attacks of gallstone pancreatitis (GSP) carry a mortality rate of 10% and a major morbidity rate of 30–40%. Most of these cases follow a mild course and are self-limited with supportive care, but approximately 20% progress to severe disease, requiring a prolonged hospital stay and intensive care, and are associated with a mortality rate approaching 30%. Three key areas in the management of patients with gallstone pancreatitis are diagnosis, risk stratification with predictors of severity and the type and timing of definitive intervention. In this chapter we have attempted to cover all relevant clinical aspects of gallstone pancreatitis regarding its etiopathogenesis, disease severity and management.

3.1 Etiopathogenesis

Considering all non-malignant gastrointestinal diseases, currently acute pancreatitis has become the most frequent reason for hospital admission. An overall mortality of 4.3% within 90 days and a 1-year mortality of 7.9% make it a lethal disease [2]. Gallstone disease is becoming more common along with heavy alcoholism as the cause of pancreatitis. Population-based studies indicate that the prevalence of gallstones in some Western countries surpasses 20% of the adult population [4].The continuous rise in gallstone prevalence is much more likely to be due to nutritional and life style factors, though genetic predisposition plays an important part in formation of gallstones [5, 6]. When a patient develops pancreatitis due to gallstones, the disease is likely to recur until the migrating bile duct stones are removed or their impaction at the duodenal papilla is prevented. According to a study involving some 5000 patients admitted with first episode of acute gallstone-associated pancreatitis, the recurrence rate was reduced from 30 to 6.7% with endoscopic sphincterotomy done during the first week; an elective interval cholecystectomy reduced it to 4.4%, and it was further reduced to 1.2% by performing endoscopic sphincterotomy combined with elective cholecystectomy during the same hospital admission [7]. The manipulation of the papilla while removing a gallstone or during a sphincterotomy, the consequent swelling can obstruct the pancreatic duct, and triggers pancreatitis in some patients. A way to address this problem is the transient insertion of small plastic stent into the pancreatic duct, which prevents the prolonged impairment of pancreatic secretion and has been shown to significantly reduce the incidence of ERCP-induced pancreatitis [8].

Taking into account the observations from various clinical and population-based studies:

a. Carrying gallstones increases the risk of developing acute pancreatitis.

b. Only gallstones that are small enough to pass through the biliary tract confer a pancreatitis risk, rather than the ones that remain asymptomatically in the gallbladder.

c. The risk of developing pancreatitis in the first place and the risk of a recurrence of pancreatitis can be reduced by strategies intended to remove the source of migrating gallstone or that prevent their impaction near the duodenal papilla.

d. Preserving the flow from the pancreatic duct is an effective way of preventing ERCP-induced pancreatitis.

3.2 Mechanisms of gallstone-induced pancreatitis

In 1856, Claude Bernard discovered that bile, when injected into the pancreatic duct of laboratory animals, can cause pancreatitis [9]. It is firmly established today that requires the passage of a gallstone from the gallbladder through the biliary tract causes initiation of pancreatitis and not gallstones, which remain in the gallbladder [10]. Eugene Opie, in 1901, postulated that impairment of the pancreatic outflow due to obstruction of the pancreatic duct causes pancreatitis [11]. Later, he modified this theory and published "common channel hypothesis," which predicted that an impacted gallstone at the papilla of Vater creates a communication between the pancreatic and the bile duct (the so-called common channel) through which bile flows into the pancreatic duct and thus causes pancreatitis (**Figure 1**).

There is inadequate experimental and clinical evidence compatible with Opie's assumptions. In fact, anatomical studies have shown that an impacted gallstone would most likely obstruct both common bile duct and pancreatic duct [12], as the communication between the pancreatic duct and the common bile duct is much too short (< 6 mm) to permit biliary reflux into the pancreatic duct [13]. The pancreatic secretory pressure is higher than biliary pressure, and pancreatic juice would flow into the bile duct rather than bile into the pancreatic duct, in the event of an existing anatomical communication between bile and pancreatic ducts [14, 15]. However, when pancreatic necrosis is firmly established, the observation of a bile-stained necrotic pancreas at the time of surgery may explain a biliopancreatic reflux due to a loss of barrier function in the damaged pancreatic duct. But this should not be regarded that biliary reflux initiates the disease process.

The "common channel" hypothesis has its own inconsistencies. In order to overcome that, it was proposed that the passage of a gallstone could damage the duodenal sphincter in a manner to cause sphincter insufficiency. This, in turn, could permit duodenal content, including bile and activated pancreatic juice, to flow through the incompetent sphincter and into the pancreatic duct [16], thus inducing pancreatitis. The perfusion of bile through the pancreatic duct has been shown to be completely harmless [17]. It has been identified that an influx of infected bile, which might occur after prolonged obstruction at the papilla, may represent an aggravating factor, as opposed to an initiating event, for the course of pancreatitis when the pressure gradient between the pancreatic duct (higher) and the bile duct (lower) is reversed [18, 19].

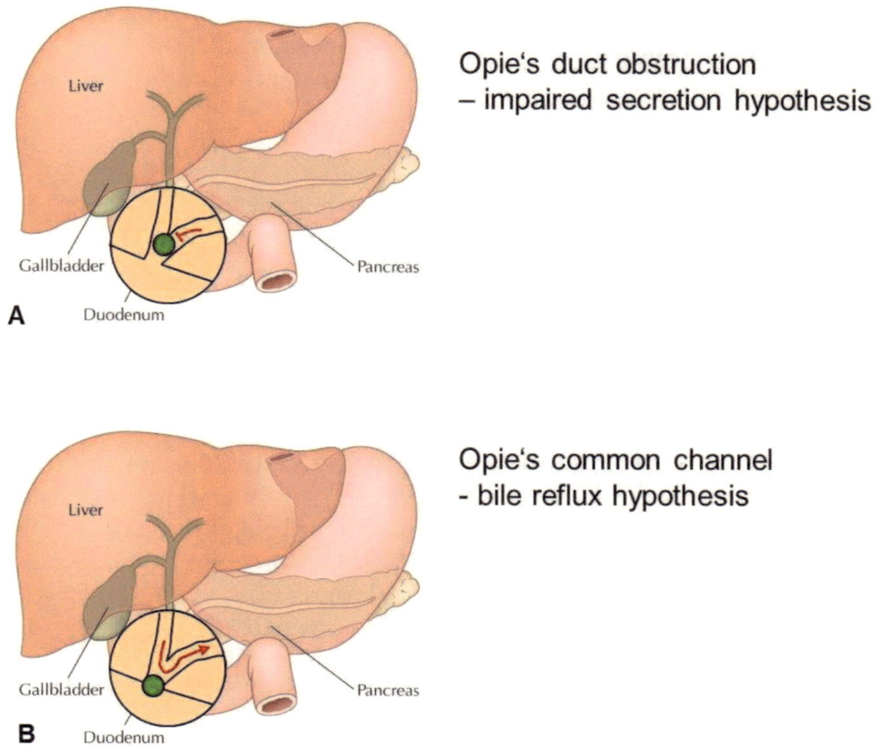

Figure 1.
The two "Opie hypotheses" for the pathogenesis of gallstone induced pancreatitis. (A) A gallstone in the biliary tract obstructs the pancreatic duct to cause an impaired flow from the exocrine pancreas triggering acinar cell or duct cell damage. Obstruction of the common bile duct is immaterial to the triggering mechanism of pancreatitis in this scenario. (B) The duodenal papilla is obstructed by an impacted gallstone, and creates a communication between the pancreatic duct and the common bile duct. This "common channel" allows passage of bile into the pancreatic duct and would trigger the onset of acute pancreatitis. Lerchand Aghdassi [23].

These data rtaken together, it is the acinar cells which are affected by the initial pathophysiological events [20] and are triggered by obstruction or impairment of flow from pancreatic duct, in accordance with Opie's initial hypothesis. Biliary reflux into pancreatic duct, by whichever mechanism, is neither required nor likely to occur during initial course of acute pancreatitis [21].

Intra-acinar pancreatic enzyme activation induces auto digestion of normal pancreatic parenchyma. As a result, acinar cells release proinflammatory cytokines, such as tumor necrosis factor-α (TNF-α) and interleukin (IL)-1, IL-2 and IL-6, and anti-inflammatory mediators, such as IL-10 and IL-1 receptor antagonist. These mediators propagate the initial injury response locally and systemically so that TNF-α, IL-1 and IL-7, neutrophils and macrophages are recruited into the pancreatic parenchyma and cause the release of more TNF- α, IL-1 and IL-6, reactive oxygen metabolites, prostaglandins, platelet-activating factor and leukotriene. The local inflammatory response increases the permeability and causes damages to the microcirculation of the pancreas further aggravating the pancreatitis. Local hemorrhage and pancreatic necrosis occur in severe cases as a result of local inflammatory response. In addition, neutrophils release some of the inflammatory mediators and aggravate the pancreatic injury by causing pancreatic enzyme activation [22].

The inflammatory cascade is self-limited in approximately 80–90% of patients. However, in the remaining patients, a vicious circle of recurring pancreatic injury and local and systemic inflammatory reaction persist. In a small number of patients, there is a massive release of inflammatory mediators to the systemic circulation.

Active neutrophils mediate acute lung injury and induce the adult respiratory distress syndrome frequently seen in patients with severe pancreatitis. The mortality seen in the early phase of pancreatitis is the result of this persistent inflammatory response.

3.3 Clinical presentation

The patients with gallstone pancreatitis usually present with acute onset of epigastric pain that radiates to back. The pain is unrelenting and accompanied typically by severe nausea and occasional vomiting. In the presence of choledocholithiasis/acute cholangitis, they have high-grade fever with chills, jaundice, acholic stools and dark urine as accompaniments.

3.4 Disease severity

In general, patients with gallstone pancreatitis can be classified into one of the three categories (mild acute pancreatitis, moderately severe acute pancreatitis and severe acute pancreatitis) according to pancreatic morphology, the presence of organ failure and local or systemic complications (**Table 1**). Morphologically as assessed by CECT, acute pancreatitis is defined as interstitial pancreatitis, which is characterized by edematous changes in the pancreatic parenchyma with or without accompanying acute peripancreatic fluid collections (APFC; **Figure 2**) or necrotizing pancreatitis with the presence of nonviable pancreatic parenchyma and, most typically, a surrounding acute necrotic collection (ANC; **Figure 3**) in the peripancreatic tissues. Organ failure in patients with gallstone pancreatitis may be transient (less than 48 h) or persistent (more than 48 h) and usually initially is accompanied by respiratory failure followed by renal failure and, in severe cases, cardiovascular failure. The Modified Marshall scoring system is being used to grade organ dysfunction by the 2012 revised Atlanta classification of acute pancreatitis, but for categorizing and managing patients with gallstone pancreatitis, the presence of transient or persistent single- or multi-organ failure is adequate. Local complications of pancreatitis are defined as an APFC, acute necrotic collection (ANC), pancreatic pseudocyst (PP) or walled-off pancreatic necrosis (WOPN). Briefly, peripancreatic fluid in the presence of interstitial edematous pancreatitis without necrosis is called an APFC, and it often

	Mild acute pancreatitis	Moderately severe pancreatitis	Severe acute pancreatitis
Morphology	Interstitial/edematous	Necrotizing	Necrotizing
SIRS response	Absent	Transient	Persistent for 1–2 weeks
Organ failure	Absent	<48 h	>48 h
Local complications			
APFC	Occasional	Often	Present initially
ANC	Absent	Occasional	Present
PP	Absent	Rare	Occasionally
WOPN	Absent	Rare	Often
Risk of infection	Nil	Low	Moderate

ANC, acute necrotic collection; APFC, acute peripancreatic fluid collection; PP, pancreatic pseudocyst; SIRS, systemic inflammatory response syndrome; WOPN, walled-off pancreatic necrosis.

Table 1.
Characteristics of the various forms of gallstone pancreatitis (2012 revised Atlanta classification).

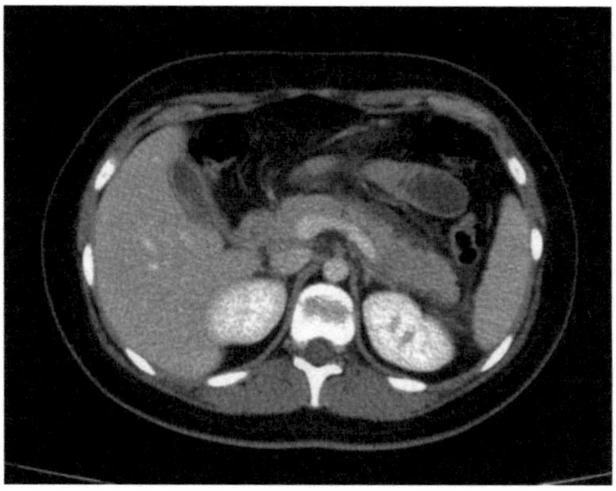

Figure 2.
APFC.

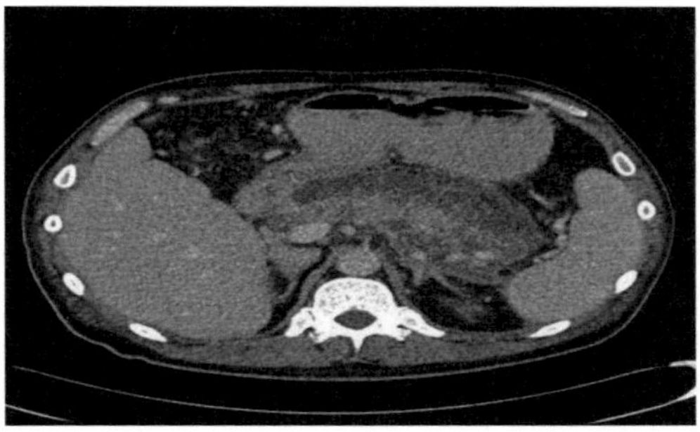

Figure 3.
WOPN.

resolves spontaneously within weeks. An ANC is a collection of fluid and necrosis associated with necrotizing pancreatitis, and it may involve the parenchyma, the peripancreatic tissues alone or both the pancreas and the retroperitoneal tissues. A pancreatic pseudocyst is an encapsulated, homogenous, enzyme-rich fluid collection with a well-defined wall that matures over 4 weeks. Finally, WOPN is a mature encapsulated collection of necrosis that develops over 4 weeks. Systemic complications of pancreatitis represent exacerbations of pre-existing comorbidities, such as coronary artery disease or chronic obstructive pulmonary disease.

3.4.1 Mild acute gallstone pancreatitis

Abdominal pain, nausea or vomiting; an increased serum amylase or lipase concentration; and transient increases in serum bilirubin, alkaline phosphatase or alanine aminotransferase concentrations characterize patients with mild acute gallstone disease. These symptoms and abnormal laboratory findings usually abate within 24–48 h. CECT is not indicated, because an APFC is not present or is not significant clinically. These findings are consistent with a gallstone or sludge which produced a transient obstruction of the pancreatic duct. The presence of gallstones is confirmed by an abdominal ultrasonography.

3.4.2 Moderately severe gallstone pancreatitis

A patient with moderately severe gallstone pancreatitis is complicated by persistent typical abdominal symptoms that may be accompanied by the presence of a fever, leukocytosis or persistently increased pancreatic- and/or liver-associated enzymes. These symptoms persist for over 48 h and may be accompanied by transient organ failure manifested by increasing oxygen requirements and an abnormally elevated creatinine or blood urine nitrogen (BUN). A CECT is indicated provided the symptoms last for more than 3 days, and that may reveal interstitial, edematous pancreatitis with an APFC or sterile pancreatic necrosis without persistent organ failure. Magnetic resonance cholangiopancreatography (MRCP) is indicated to confirm or exclude the presence of an obstructing stone in patients with continually increased liver-associated enzymes (bilirubin >4) which may have biliary obstruction from gallstones.

3.4.3 Severe acute gallstone pancreatitis

Patients with severe acute gallstone pancreatitis have severe abdominal symptoms and develop persistent single or multiple organ failure. These patients exhibit signs of the systemic inflammatory response syndrome with tachycardia, hypothermia or hyperthermia, leukocytosis and tachypnea. They require admission to the intensive care unit and often require intubation and mechanical ventilation, renal replacement therapy and/or inotropic support due to progressive organ failure. After resuscitation and stabilization, CECT may demonstrate pancreatic necrosis with local complications; however, necrotizing pancreatitis evolves over days and weeks, and early CECT may not demonstrate significant pancreatic or peripancreatic findings. Patients with high suspicion of acute cholangitis require evaluation with MRCP, and perhaps, in these critically ill patients, the most efficient procedure for the relief of biliary obstruction is endoscopic retrograde cholangiopancreatography (ERCP).

3.5 Diagnosis

A definitive diagnosis of acute pancreatitis requires two of the following three criteria:

(1) Abdominal pain that is constant, severe, epigastric and often radiating to the back; accompanied by nausea, vomiting and anorexia; and exacerbated by oral intake; (2) serum lipase (or amylase) level at least three times the upper limit of normal; and (3) characteristic imaging findings, ideally with a contrast-enhanced computed tomography (CT). It is often advisable to delay CT for 72 h, in patients with typical abdominal pain and elevated lipase or amylase, and at that time to perform a dedicated pancreas protocol CT (PPCT) with an early arterial phase and a delayed portal venous phase, ideally calibrated to cardiac output. Important advantages of this 72-hour delay in the PPCT include avoiding excessive radiation and contrast exposure associated with repeat CT imaging, allowing free fluid to begin to coalesce and increasing the ability to distinguish pancreatic necrosis from transiently ischemic areas. In some cases of obviously mild pancreatitis, or frequently recurrent alcoholic pancreatitis, CT may be omitted.

The diagnosis of gallstones as the cause of the pancreatitis is largely a diagnosis of exclusion. Careful history-taking is essential for patients who have acute pancreatitis to help rule out non gallstone causes. In addition, several different laboratory values, such as elevated aminotransferases, bilirubin and alkaline phosphatase, are useful in identifying a biliary origin of pancreatitis. Initial imaging with ultrasound (US) is essential to confirm the presence of gallstones or sludge and to measure the diameter of the common bile duct. Although the US is optimally 95% sensitive in detecting cholelithiasis, in gallstone pancreatitis, the sensitivity may decrease to

	Finding	**Points**	
Grade	A: Normal pancreas	1	
	B: Pancreatic enlargement	2	
	C: Pancreatic or peripancreatic inflammation	3	
	D: Single peripancreatic fluid collection	4	
	E: Two or more fluid collections or peripancreatic air	5	
Necrosis	<30%	2	
	30–50%	4	
	>50%	6	
CT severity index	**0–3 (%)**	**4–6 (%)**	**7–10 (%)**
Morbidity	8	35	92
Morality	3	6	17

Table 2.
Computer tomography severity index (Balthazar score).

60% from 80% because of the increased bowel gas caused by concomitant ileus. A CECT with pancreatic protocol is indicated in patients with moderate and severe pancreatitis, ideally 48–72 h after diagnosis, and may demonstrate pancreatic necrosis with local complications (**Table 2**).

3.6 Treatment

In acute gallstone pancreatitis, intravenous fluid resuscitation is the mainstay of treatment regardless of disease severity. All patients require frequent serial re-evaluations because even patients with apparently mild disease may go on to rapidly develop severe pancreatitis and require intensive care, which may include mechanical ventilation and cardiovascular support.

3.6.1 Mild-moderate disease

The initial fluid administration should be in boluses followed by titration of infusion based on urine output, heart rate, blood pressure and correction of acidemia. Oral intake may be restricted in these patients on presentation but should begin soon after, as tolerated, typically within 24 h. If nausea and vomiting persist, however, nasogastric tube decompression can protect against vomiting and aspiration. While this treatment is going on, the primary complaint of the patient is to be addressed, which is severe abdominal pain. This is taken care of mainly by intravenous opiates. There is no role for prophylactic antibiotics unless an infection has been identified. However those patients with cholangitis and those who go on to develop extensive necrotizing pancreatitis, intravenous antibiotics may be warranted. Patients with significant cholangitis in addition to gallstone pancreatitis require urgent ERCP. Some people advocate early routine ERCP for all patients, but the latest guidelines limit ERCP and sphincterotomy to those patients with severe disease, to decrease complications.

Patients with moderately severe gallstone pancreatitis have evidence of local complications from pancreatic injury and transient organ failure and thus should be managed in a monitored setting. Because organ failure is transient with this condition, rapid improvement is anticipated, and a prolonged intensive care unit stay should be unnecessary.

However, the duration of hospitalization may be dependent on the local complications related to pancreatic injury. Edematous pancreatitis with an APFC should resolve relatively quickly, whereas sterile necrosis may cause persistent symptoms and limit per oral intake, necessitating institution of enteral nutrition. For patients who have sterile necrosis, follow-up CECT is recommended to ensure resolution of the pancreatic injury without complicating features such as the development of a pancreatic pseudocyst.

Laparoscopic cholecystectomy should be offered to patients with mild GSP during the index hospitalization, generally as soon as the patient is stable with significant resolution of acute symptoms.

3.6.2 Severe disease

Patient with severe disease should be treated aggressively in a higher center with well-equipped intensive care units, endoscopy and operative rooms all of which are staffed by critical care experts, gastroenterologists, interventional radiologists and surgeons. These patients develop a profound SIRS response and often have rapid deterioration requiring intubation and mechanical ventilation, renal replacement therapy and inotropic support. This critical period is driven by cytokine response and may last for 1–2 weeks. Aggressive fluid resuscitation is the cornerstone of initial therapy in severe. The goals of therapy during this period of critical illness include maintenance of oxygen delivery to the central nervous system and viscera by mechanical ventilation, adequate resuscitation with Lactated Ringer's solution, inotropic administration as needed to support blood pressure and decrease heart rate, maintenance of renal function with or without renal replacement therapy and nutritional support. Enteral nutrition should be tried, though less often possible, because of less incidence of infected pancreatic necrosis. Antibiotics are often used to prevent conversion of sterile necrosis to infected necrosis, if the necrosis is <30%.

As the systemic inflammatory response wanes over 1–2 weeks, these patients will develop local complications of necrotizing pancreatitis. An early ERCP plus sphincterotomy along with conservative management can help decrease complications of severe disease. By 4–6 weeks these complications mature and management to be guided according to symptoms. Unlike in mild disease, an early operation should be avoided in severe pancreatitis, whether for cholecystectomy or pancreatic debridement. There are, however, a few notable exceptions, such as abdominal compartment syndrome, refractory hemorrhage and colonic necrosis or perforation, in which case immediate operation is warranted.

An ANC accompanying pancreatic necrosis may be sterile or infected. Sterile necrosis often requires no intervention, and patients recover over time except for the infrequent patient who develops failure-to-thrive syndrome as a result of sterile necrosis. Patients with failure-to-thrive syndrome may require percutaneous drainage or endoscopic or operative debridement for full recovery. Those patients with infected necrosis require drainage and debridement of infected pancreatic tissues with vigorous antibiotic therapy. The mode of drainage or debridement can vary from percutaneous drainage, endoscopic or laparoscopic debridement to dual-modality drainage (combined percutaneous and endoscopic drainage). The open surgical approaches are heterogenous, and some of these approaches are no longer used in contemporary management.

Importantly, before debridement, a CECT should be obtained to ascertain the presence of the disconnected pancreatic duct syndrome. A viable pancreatic remnant in the tail separated by a substantial area of pancreatic necrosis in the neck of the gland should lead to the suspicion of a disconnected pancreas. This warrants the need for distal pancreatectomy and splenectomy accompanied by pancreatic debridement as necessary, regardless of the surgical approach. Finally, concomitant with or following pancreatic drainage or debridement, the patient must have a cholecystectomy to prevent further episodes of gallstone-induced pancreatitis. The outcomes of patients with severe acute gallstone pancreatitis are variable depending on the patient's overall condition, the extent of the disease, the type of procedure performed, the expertise of the providers and the institutional experience with such patients.

4. Conclusion

Acute gallstone pancreatitis represents a wide spectrum of disease ranging from mild disease that resolves spontaneously to severe disease with SIRS and necrotizing pancreatitis. These patients are best managed by a multidisciplinary approach to combat complications. Finally they should have a timely cholecystectomy to treat the cause of disease.

Author details

Sam Koruth* and Sooraj Sankar
Lourdes Hospital, Kochi, India

*Address all correspondence to: koruth.sam@gmail.com

References

[1] Peery AF, Dellon ES, Lund J, Crockett SD, McGowan CE, Bulsiewicz WJ, et al. Burden of gastrointestinal disease in the United States: 2012 update. Gastroenterology. 2012;**143**(5):1179-1187

[2] Hazra N, Gulliford M. Evaluating pancreatitis in primary care: A population-based cohort study. The British Journal of General Practice. 2014;**64**(622):e295-e301

[3] Cushieri A, Dubois F, Mouiel J, Mouret P, Becker H, Buess G, et al. The European experience with laparoscopic cholecystectomy. American Journal of Surgery. 1991;**161**:385-387

[4] Volzke H, Baumeister SE, Alte D, Hoffmann W, Schwahn C, Simon P, et al. Independent risk factors for gallstone formation in a region with high cholelithiasis prevalence. Digestion. 2005;**71**(2):97-105

[5] von Kampen O, Buch S, Nothnagel M, Azocar L, Molina H, Brosch M, et al. Genetic and functional identification of the likely causative variant for cholesterol gallstone disease at the ABCG5/8 lithogenic locus. Hepatology. 2013;**57**(6):2407-2417

[6] Buch S, Schafmayer C, Volzke H, Seeger M, Miquel JF, Sookoian SC, et al. Loci from a genome-wide analysis of bilirubin levels are associated with gallstone risk and composition. Gastroenterology. 2010;**139**(6):1942-1951 e1942

[7] Mustafa A, Begaj I, Deakin M, Durkin D, Corless DJ, Wilson R, et al. Long-term effectiveness of cholecystectomy and endoscopic sphincterotomy in the management of gallstone pancreatitis. Surgical Endoscopy. 2014;**28**(1):127-133

[8] Fan JH, Qian JB, Wang YM, Shi RH, Zhao CJ. Updated meta-analysis of pancreatic stent placement in preventing post-endoscopic retrograde cholangiopancreatography pancreatitis. World Journal of Gastroenterology. 2015;**21**(24):7577-7583

[9] Bernard C. Lecons de physiologie experimentale. Vol. 2. Paris: Bailliere; 1856. p. 758

[10] Acosta JM, Ledesma CL. Gallstone migration as a cause of acute pancreatitis. The New England Journal of Medicine. 1974;**290**(9):484-487

[11] Opie E. The relation of cholelithiasis to disease of the pancreas and to fat necrosis. Johns Hopkins Hospital Bulletin. 1901;**12**:19-21

[12] Mann FC, Giordano AS. The bile factor in pancreatitis. Archives of Surgery. 1923;**6**:1-30

[13] DiMagno EP, Shorter RG, Taylor WF, Go VL. Relationships between pancreaticobiliary ductal anatomy and pancreatic ductal and parenchymal histology. Cancer. 1982;**49**(2):361-368

[14] Carr-Locke DL, Gregg JA. Endoscopic manometry of pancreatic and biliary sphincter zones in man. Basal results in healthy volunteers. Digestive Diseases and Sciences. 1981;**26**(1):7-15

[15] McCutcheon AD. Reflux of duodenal contents in the pathogenesis of pancreatitis. Gut. 1964;**5**:260-265

[16] Menguy RB, Hallenbeck GA, Bollman JL, Grindlay JH. Intraductal pressures and sphincteric resistance in canine pancreatic and biliary ducts after various stimuli. Surgery, Gynecology & Obstetrics. 1958;**106**(3):306-320

[17] Robinson TM, Dunphy JE. Continuous perfusion of bile and

protease activators through the pancreas. JAMA. 1963;**183**:530-533

[18] Arendt T, Nizze H, Monig H, Kloehn S, Stuber E, Folsch UR. Biliary pancreatic reflux- induced acute pancreatitis--myth or possibility? European Journal of Gastroenterology & Hepatology. 1999;**11**(3):329-335

[19] Csendes A, Sepulveda A, Burdiles P, Braghetto I, Bastias J, Schutte H, et al. Common bile duct pressure in patients with common bile duct stones with or without acute suppurative cholangitis. Archives of Surgery. 1988;**123**(6):697-699

[20] Lerch MM, Saluja AK, Dawra R, Ramarao P, Saluja M, Steer ML. Acute necrotizing pancreatitis in the opossum: Earliest morphological changes involve acinar cells. Gastroenterology. 1992;**103**(1):205-213

[21] Pohle T, Konturek JW, Domschke W, Lerch MM. Spontaneous flow of bile through the human pancreatic duct in the absence of pancreatitis: Nature's human experiment. Endoscopy. 2003;**35**(12):1072-1075

[22] Elfar M, Gaber LW, Sabek O, et al. The inflammatory cascade in acute pancreatitis: Relevance to clinical disease. The Surgical Clinics of North America. 2007;**87**:1325-1340

[23] Lerch MM, Aghdassi A. Gallstone-Related Pathogenesis Of Acute Pancreatitis. Version 1.0, August 19, 2016

Chapter 7

Gall Bladder Carcinoma: Clinical Presentations and Different Modalities of Treatment

Wala Ben Kridis, Nabil Toumi, Jamel Daoud, Afef Khanfir and Mounir Frikha

Abstract

Gallbladder cancer (GBC) is the most common cancer of the biliary tract and has a particularly high incidence in Chile, Japan and northern India. The clinical presentation of GBC is often vague or delayed relative to pathologic progression, contributing to advanced staging and dismal prognosis at the time of diagnosis. In the diagnosis of GBC, differential diagnosis and determination of the local extension of tumor are important. For these purposes, imaging modalities such as endoscopic ultrasonography (EUS), CT, MRI and magnetic resonance cholangio-pancreatography (MRCP) are useful. The treatment of localized GBC is based on surgery. Chemotherapy has been used extensively in advanced GBC, and we have gained some experience with gemcitabine-based combination (with cisplatin and oxaliplatin or with capecitabine) regimens.

Keywords: gallbladder carcinoma, clinical presentation, treatment

1. Introduction

Biliary tract cancers (BTCs) are invasive adenocarcinomas that arise from the epithelial lining of the gallbladder and intrahepatic and extrahepatic (hilar and distal common bile duct) bile ducts. Gallbladder cancer (GBC) is one of the most common malignant tumors of the extrahepatic bile ducts with high incidence in Japan, Chile and northern India [1]. The incidence of GBC steadily increases with age. Women are affected two to six times more often than men, with predominance in whites. Several risk factors are incriminated in the occurrence of this malignant tumor, and the main one is gallstone disease. The symptomatology is varied and nonspecific, dominated mainly by the pain of the right hypochondrium, which poses a problem of early diagnosis and management. The circumstances of discovery are multiple: preoperative, intraoperative and postoperative. GBC is characterized by local extension, regional lymph node metastases and distant metastases. Usually, GBC is the most aggressive of the biliary cancers with the shortest overall survival [1]. Complete surgical resection is the only chance for cure. However, only 10% of patients are considered surgical candidates [1]. Among patients who undergo curative resection, recurrence rates are high. Patients with unresectable or metastatic GBC have a very poor prognosis.

2. Epidemiology

Gallbladder cancer is the most common cancer of the bile ducts. It accounts for 3% of all malignant tumors and ranks fifth among digestive cancers after cancer of the colon, rectum, stomach and pancreas [2].

The incidence rates are high in Asia and Latin America, relatively high in some countries in eastern and central Europe, yet low in the United States and most Western and Mediterranean European countries [3]. Gallbladder cancer tends to afflict indigenous populations, according to a vast global cancer registry on five continents (representing 704.4 million people or 11% of the world population) [4]. Mapuche Indians from Valdivia, Chile and South America exhibit the highest rate of gallbladder cancer: 12.3/100,000 for males and 27.3/100,000 for females. American Indians in New Mexico, USA, follow with an average annual rate of 8.9/100,000. For these native people, GBC mortality rates exceed those for breast (8.7/100,000), cervical (8.0/100,000), pancreatic (7.4/100,000) and ovarian cancers (7.3/100,000) [5]. According to the literature, the sex ratio women-men ranges from 2:1 to 3:1. In India and South America, the sex ratio is particularly very high: 5/1 to 6/1. However, this difference between the two sexes is less pronounced in East Asia, where the sex ratio between men and women [6]. Gallbladder cancer rates tend to increase with advancing age. The median age was 67 years in a Memorial Sloan-Kettering report of 435 gallbladder cancer patients [7]. Gallbladder cancer is found in 1–2% of cholecystectomized patients. It is suggested that the presence of vesicular calculus may cause dysplasia of the vesicular mucosa after chronic irritation.

Usually, gallbladder cancer develops over 5–15 years, when metaplasia progresses to dysplasia, carcinoma in situ and, then, invasive cancer. Only 10% of patients are resectable at the time of surgery [6] with high recurrence rates [8].

3. Diagnosis

3.1 Symptoms and signs of gallbladder carcinoma

The clinical presentation of GBC is often vague or delayed relative to pathologic progression, contributing to advanced staging and dismal prognosis at the time of diagnosis. The clinical presentation is nonspecific. Pain is the most constant symptom. It is present in 72–77% of patients [9]. Frequently, it is an intense paroxysmal pain with respiratory inhibition, sitting in the right hypochondrium, and with posterior irradiation to the tip of the right shoulder blade and anterior to the right shoulder, realizing the classic pain in sling. It could be atypical such as epigastralgia and diffuse abdominal pain [9].

Jaundice is observed in 58% of cases. It may be secondary to either tumor invasion or extrinsic compression of the bile ducts by lymphadenopathy or tumor or by the presence of liver metastases [10]. Nausea and vomiting are found in 20–49% of cases. Clinical examination may be strictly normal at the early stages. The most common signs are evidence of a very advanced disease. GBC is manifested in 15–50% of cases by a mass of the right hypochondrium [11]. Abdominal palpation shows a sensitivity of the right hypochondrium in 50–80% of cases [11]. A defense of the right hypochondrium or even a positive sign of Murphy can be found on the examination, but they remain an unspecific signs [11].

3.2 Diagnosis

Imaging modalities such as ultrasonography (US), endoscopic ultrasonography (EUS), computed tomography (CT), *magnetic resonance imaging* (MRI) and magnetic resonance cholangiopancreatography (MRCP) are useful. EUS has good sensitivity in differentiating benign gallbladder diseases from GBC [12]. CT and MRI examinations are useful for local and metastatic staging [13].

Ultrasonography is the first examination to be carried out in the diagnostic approach in front of a patient presenting a biliary symptomatology or for the preoperative study of a vesicular tumor (**Figure 1**, [14, 15]). It has a sensitivity of 85% and a specificity of 80% in the diagnosis of tumors of the gallbladder. Budding image is the most common image [15]. It is a vegetative lesion projecting into the vesicular lumen. It can be single or multiple and is manifested by a hypo or iso-echoic image without shadow cone, irregular edge and implantation base. EUS allows directly visualizing the tumor and evaluating its deep extension in the vesicular wall, in the hepatic parenchyma and the bile ducts [14]. It also makes it possible to differentiate an early tumor from an advanced tumor. It has a significant sensitivity for the etiological diagnosis of neoplastic icterus.

If US suggest a resectable GBC, CT, MRI with magnetic resonance cholangiography (MRC) and/or traditional cholangiography often provide additional information [16]. These modalities allowed specific staging [17].

CT is to be done in second intension after the ultrasound. It allows the diagnosis of GBC in 60–74% of cases. However, its main interest lies in the establishment of the tumor extension report. The CT scan aspects are similar to those detected by ultrasound. A parietal thickening (**Figure 2**) or a budding tumor presenting as a hypodense, heterogeneous lesion containing hypodense zones and other hyperdense secondary to tumor necrosis may be found. The enhancement by the tumor may be diffuse or partial, preferentially, peripheral in case of avascular central necrosis [18, 19]. Although CT is inferior to ultrasound in depicting mucosal irregularity, mural thickening and cholelithiasis, it is superior for evaluating the thickness of portions of the gallbladder wall that are obscured by gallstones or mural calcification on ultrasound. In unclear cases, hybrid PET-CT systems may provide structural and functional information simultaneously and may offer early and accurate staging with high specificity [20].

The GBC appears hypo- or isosignal in T1 and hypersignal in T2 at MRI, the perilesional inflammation in hypersignal T2 and the calculations are hyposignal. Intravenous gadolinium injection increases sensitivity and provides additional data

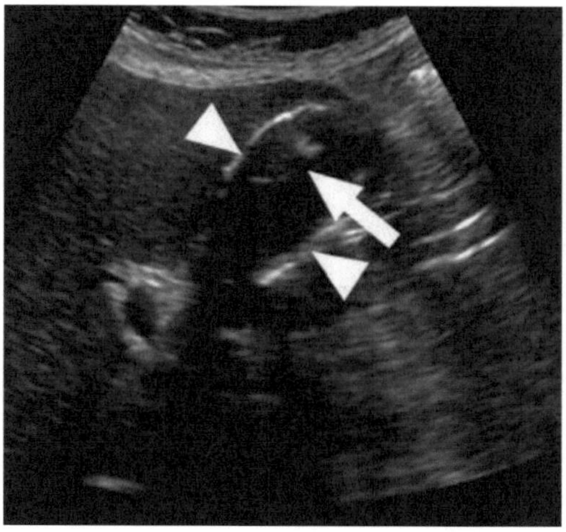

Figure 1.
Ultrasonography shows hyperechoic shadowing portions of gallbladder wall (arrowheads) consistent with porcelain gallbladder and hypoechoic, polypoid mass (arrow) suggestive of malignant degeneration into gallbladder carcinoma.

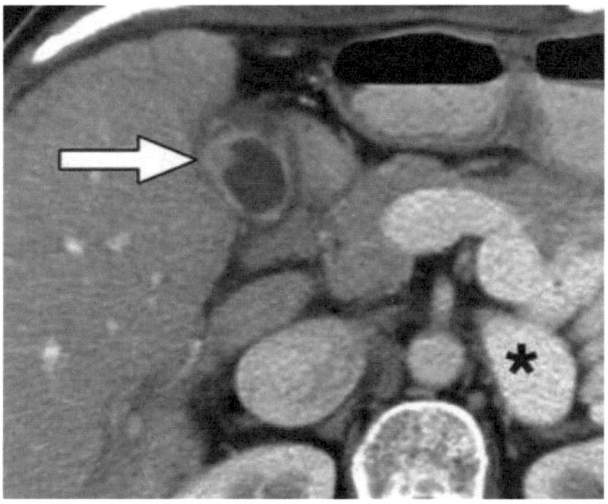

Figure 2.
Contrast-enhanced CT scan during portal venous phase shows focal nodular thickening (arrow) and diffuse gallbladder wall thickening.

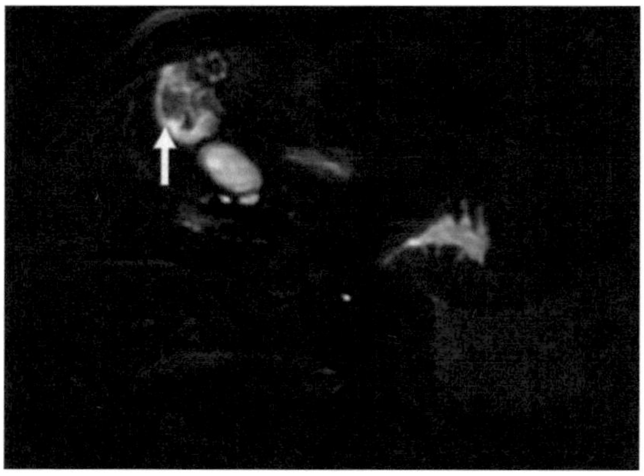

Figure 3.
Axial fat-saturated T2 fast spin image shows a mildly hyperintense, polypoidal and intraluminal gallbladder mass (arrow).

Extension		**M0**			**M1**
		N0	**N1***	**N2****	
Tis	Carcinoma in situ	0	—	—	—
T1a	Tumor invades the lamina propria	I	IIIB		IVB
T1b	Tumor invades the muscular layer				
T2	Tumor invades the perimuscular connective tissue; no extension beyond the serosa or into the liver	II			
T3	Tumor perforates the serosa and/or invades the liver and/ or other adjacent organ or extrahepatic bile ducts	IIIA			
T4	Tumor invades the main portal vein or the hepatic artery or two or more extrahepatic organs	IVA			

**Along the cystic duct, the common hepatic duct, the common hepatic artery and the portal vein.*
***Peri-aortic, peri-cellar, celiac trunk and superior mesenteric artery.*

Table 1.
TNM classification (7th edition).

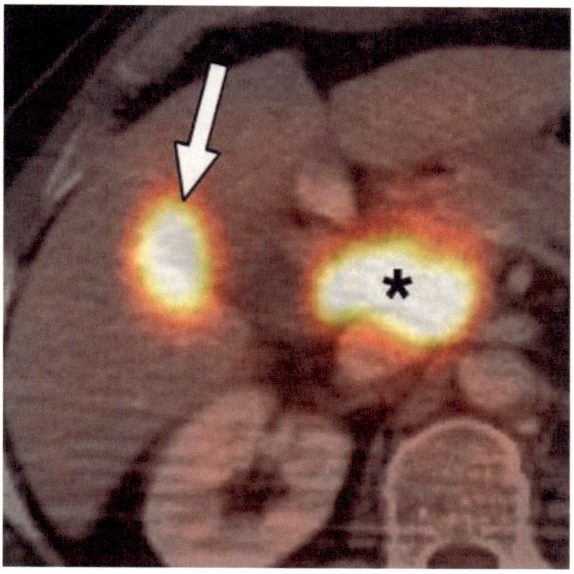

Figure 4.
PET/CT image: gallbladder carcinoma (arrow) with lymph nodes (asterisk).

on vascular involvement (**Figure 3**). The section thickness should be 5 mm or less, with a 1–2 mm gap between sections.

Cholangio-MRI is a very useful test for jaundice. It allows to specify the tumor extension. It may be the only examination to be performed after ultrasound in patients with jaundice. Dynamic MRI with MRCP is an accurate and a reliable method of showing GBC and in assessing its local and regional extent as part of preoperative assessment [13]. However, only the pathological study could confirm the diagnosis of gallbladder carcinoma.

In unclear cases, fluorodeoxyglucose-positron emission tomography (FDG-PET) can be considered to establish the benign or the malignant nature of the lesion and to obtain a primary staging study (**Figure 4**).

Table 1 showed TNM classification (7th edition)—UICC—AJCC (2010) cancers of gall bladder.

4. Treatment

4.1 Localized GCC

4.1.1 Surgery

4.1.1.1 Tis, T1a, T1b and T2 cancers discovered incidentally on the cholecystectomy

The reference is IVb-V bisegmentectomy with lymph node dissection and possibly resection of the bile duct. Bisegmentectomy can be discussed in favor of resection of the vesicular bed for these "small cancers," especially if the cancer is located on the free side of the gallbladder. Similarly, resection of the bile duct is recommended only in cases of cystic involvement or patent nodal invasion (**Figure 5**) [21].

Systematic secondary resection of trocar orifices is currently controversial.

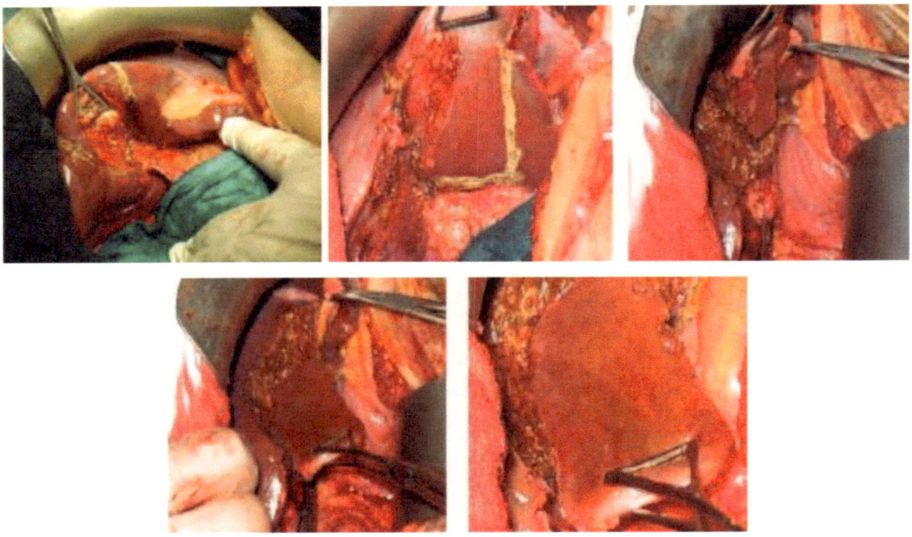

Figure 5.
Photos d'une bi-segmentectomy IVb-V.

4.1.1.2 Locally advanced tumors >T2

The extent of liver resection remains controversial. Thus, an IVb-V bisegmentectomy or a more extensive hepatic resection of the trisegmentectomy type may be proposed, and for tumors invading the hepatic pedicle, an enlarged right hepatectomy or a central hepatectomy (IV, V, VIII) associated with a segment I resection. Segment I resection is especially useful for tumors invading the hepatic hilum. Direct invasion of the colon, duodenum or liver is not an absolute contraindication to resection, but the morbidity and mortality of these combined resections are high. Ganglion dissection should include extensive resection of the hepatic pedicle ganglia, anterior and posterior pancreatic ganglia and peeling of the hepatic artery until birth in the celiac trunk. Some authors recommend extensive curling, extended to the celiac trunk, to the trunk of the superior mesenteric artery down the anterior aspect of the aorta (para-aortic ganglia). Involvement of the hepatic pedicle and the main bile duct is early in gallbladder cancer without necessarily having a clinical impact (jaundice) or contact with the tumor [22]. In addition, removal of the main bile duct facilitates nodal dissection of the hepatic pedicle. It is therefore recommended for tumors >T2.

4.1.1.3 Palliative surgery

Surgical biliary shunts (and trans-tumor intubations) have not been demonstrated superior to prosthetic drainage in terms of quality of life or survival time. Their mortality (>25% in several series) and their morbidity are not negligible. However, the surgical biliary drainage usually allows prolonged palliation to the entire survival patients [22].

4.1.2 Adjuvant treatment

The role of adjuvant chemoradiotherapy is not well defined because of a lack of randomized trials. Most of the published studies are retrospective with small numbers of patients and a mix of gallbladder and bile duct tumors.

A systematic review and meta-analysis of published data from 20 studies between 1960 and 2010 (6712 patients) showed a nonsignificant improvement in overall survival with any adjuvant therapy (chemotherapy (CT), radiotherapy (RT) or radiochemotherapy (RCT)) compared to curative surgery alone (HR 0.74, p = 0.06). There was no difference between gall bladder tumors and bile duct tumors (p = 0.68). The association became significant when both cancer registries were excluded, with a significantly higher benefit of CT or RCT than RT alone (OR: 0.39, 0.61 and 0.98, respectively, p = 0.02). The greatest benefit of adjuvant treatments was observed with N+ status (OR: 0.49, p = 0.004) or R1 (OR: 0.36, p = 0.002) [23]. There is no randomized trial of adjuvant RT or RCT. However, there are only heterogeneous retrospective series, addressing the issue of adjuvant radiation therapy. In these small series, differences in patient selection criteria, staging systems, extent of resections, radiation therapy techniques and doses and chemotherapy schedules, it is difficult to pinpoint the exact role of adjuvant therapy in GBC [24, 25]. Bilcap study is a phase III study that included patients with completely resected cholangiocarcinoma (CCA) or gallbladder cancer (including liver and pancreatic resection, as appropriate), with adequate biliary drainage, no ongoing infection, adequate renal, hematological and liver function and ECOG PS ≤ 2. It demonstrated that capecitabine improved overall survival when used as adjuvant and should become standard of care [26].

4.2 Metastatic GCC

A small Scandinavian randomized controlled trial showed that a chemotherapy by 5Fluorouracil and (more etoposide so good general condition) increased the quality of life and survival compared exclusive supportive care in patients with advanced pancreatic or biliary cancer (6.0 vs. 2.5 months, p < 0.01), however not significantly in the patient subgroup with biliary cancer, and at the cost of considerable toxicity (grade 3–4, 41%) [27]. A single-center Indian randomized controlled trial in 81 patients with carcinoma of the gallbladder has shown a global survival benefit of chemotherapy by gemcitabine and oxaliplatin not only compared to exclusive supportive care but also compared to a chemotherapy with 5FU and folinic acid (9.5, 4.5 and 4.6 months respectively, p = 0.039) [28]. Collectively, these two trials show that first-line chemotherapy is legitimate in patients with advanced biliary cancer whose general condition is not too impaired (PS 0–2).

The British randomized controlled trial ABC-02 demonstrated, in 410 patients with PS ECOG 0–2 (ECOG 0–1: 88%) and controlled biliary obstruction (total bilirubinemia <1.5 N), superiority of gemcitabine-cisplatin combination (GEMCIS regimen) on gemcitabine alone (survival overall: 11.7 vs. 8.1 months, hazard ratio [HR]: 0.64 [95% CI, 0.52–0.80], p < 0.001) [29]. The benefit of survival with the GEMCIS regimen was independent not only of tumor stage (locally advanced or metastatic) but also of the primary tumor site (intra- or extrahepatic bile ducts, hile, gallbladder, vater bulb). These results were supported by those of the randomized trial Phase II Japanese BT-22 in 84 patients (ECOG 0-1: 100%) [30]. These results make the GEMCIS regimen the first standard of first-line chemotherapy in patients with advanced biliary cancer. The GEMOX scheme [31] is an alternative, despite the lack of a randomized controlled trial comparing these two regimens. The treatment of metastatic forms is to be discussed according to the general condition (PS, age). In case of PS > 2, it is recommended to do exclusive support care. In case of PS between 0 and 2, it is the indication of a palliative CT by gemcitabine-cisplatin. The GEMOX scheme is an alternative.

5. Conclusion

GBC represents a major challenge in oncology. The only curative treatment for this disease is surgical resection. The roles of radiation and chemoradiation in the neoadjuvant and adjuvant settings remain to be defined in prospective studies. Bilcap study demonstrated that capecitabine improved overall survival in adjuvant situation. The treatment of metastatic forms is to be discussed according to the general condition (PS, age). In case of PS > 2, it is recommended to do exclusive support care. For patients with PS between 0 and 2, it is the indication of a palliative CT by gemcitabine-cisplatin. The GEMOX scheme represents an alternative.

Conflict of interest

None.

Author details

Wala Ben Kridis[1*], Nabil Toumi[1], Jamel Daoud[2], Afef Khanfir[1] and Mounir Frikha[1]

1 Department of Oncology, Habib Bourguiba Hospital, Sfax, Tunisia

2 Department of Radiotherapy, Habib Bourguiba Hospital, Sfax, Tunisia

*Address all correspondence to: walabenkridis@yahoo.fr

References

[1] Kiran RP, Pokala N, Dudrick SJ. Incidence pattern and survival for gallbladder cancer over three decades—An analysis of 10301 patients. Annals of Surgical Oncology. 2007;**14**:827-832

[2] Lazcano-Ponce EC, Miquel JF, Muñoz N, et al. Epidemiology and molecular pathology of gallbladder cancer. CA: A Cancer Journal for Clinicians. 2001;**51**(6):349-364

[3] Levy AD, Murakata LA, Rohrmann CA Jr. Gallbladder carcinoma: Radiologic-pathologic correlation. Radiographics. 2001;**21**(2):295-314. Questionnaire, 549–555

[4] Curado MP, Edwards B, Shin HR, et al., editors. Cancer Incidence in Five Continents, Vol. IX. Lyon: International Agency for Research on Cancer; 2007

[5] Surveillance, Epidemiology and End-Results Program (SEER). The Four Most Common Cancers for Different Ethnic Populations 2013. Bethesda, MD: National Cancer Institute; 2013

[6] Sheth S, Bedford A, Chopra S. Primary gallbladder cancer: Recognition of risk factors and the role of prophylactic cholecystectomy. The American Journal of Gastroenterology. 2000;**95**(6):1402-1410

[7] Duffy A, Capanu M, Abou-Alfa GK, et al. Gallbladder cancer (GBC): 10 year experience at Memorial Sloan-Kettering Cancer Centre (MSKCC). Journal of Surgical Oncology. 2008;**98**(7):485-489

[8] Randi G, Franceschi S, La Vecchia C. Gallbladder cancer worldwide: Geographical distribution and risk factors. International Journal of Cancer. 2006;**118**(7):1591-1602

[9] van der Horst MP, Hendriks ER, Blok P, Brouwers MA, Steup WH. Diversity of complaints in manifesting carcinoma of the gallbladder. Nederlands Tijdschrift voor Geneeskunde. 2007;**151**:1083-1086

[10] von Meyenfeldt EM, Mantel SF, Gouma DJ, van Gulik TM. Tumors in the gallbladder: A possible differentiation between malignant and benign tumours. Nederlands Tijdschrift voor Geneeskunde. 2007;**151**:1049-1054

[11] Furlan A, Ferris JV, Hosseinzadeh K, Borhani AA. Gallbladder carcinoma update: Multimodality imaging evaluation, staging, and treatment options. American Journal of Roentgenology. 2008;**191**:1440-1447

[12] Vialle R, Velasco S, Milin S, Bricot V, Richer JP, Levillain PM, et al. Imaging in the diagnosis and the staging of gallbladder tumors. Gastroentérologie Clinique et Biologique. 2008;**32**:931-941

[13] Samad A. Gall bladder carcinoma in patients undergoing cholecystectomy for cholelithiasis. The Journal of the Pakistan Medical Association. 2005;**55**:497-499

[14] Gore RM, Shelhamer RP. Biliary tract neoplasms: Diagnosis and staging. Cancer Imaging. 2007;**7**:S15-S23

[15] Matsubara S, Arizumi T, Togawa O, Sasaki T, Yamamoto N, Nakai Y, et al. Endoscopic transpapillary approach to the gallbladder for diagnosing gallbladder cancer. Canadian Journal of Gastroenterology. 2007;**21**:809-813

[16] Oikarinen H. Diagnostic imaging of carcinomas of the gallbladder and the bile ducts. Acta Radiologica. 2006;**47**:345-358

[17] Ching BH, Yeh BM, Westphalen AC, Joe BN, Qayyum A, Coakley FV. CT differentiation of adenomyomatosis and gallbladder cancer. American Journal of Roentgenology. 2007;**189**:62-66

[18] Maldjian PD, Ghesani N, Ahmed S, Liu Y. Adenomyomatosis of the gallbladder: Another cause for a "hot" gallbladder on 18F-FDG PET. American Journal of Roentgenology. 2007;**189**:W36-W38

[19] Rodríguez-Fernández A, Gómez-Río M, Medina-Benítez A, Moral JV, Ramos-Font C, Ramia-Angel JM, et al. Application of modern imaging methods in diagnosis of gallbladder cancer. Journal of Surgical Oncology. 2006;**93**:650-664

[20] Ben Farhat L, Askri A, Jeribi R, Daly N, Hendaoui L. CT evaluation of locoregional spread of carcinoma of the gallbladder. Journal de Chirurgie. 2009;**146**:34-39

[21] Ito H, Ito K, D'Angelica M, et al. Accurate staging for gallbladder cancer: Implications for surgical therapy and pathological assessment. Annals of Surgery. 2011;**254**:320-325

[22] Shimizu Y, Ohtsuka M, Ito H, et al. Should the extrahepatic bile duct be resected for locally advanced gallbladder cancer? Surgery. 2004;**136**:1012-1017

[23] Horgan AM, Amir E, Walter T, Knox JJ. Adjuvant therapy in the treatment of biliary tract cancer: A systematic review and meta-analysis. Journal of Clinical Oncology. 2012;**30**:1934-1940

[24] Ben-Josef E, Guthrie KA, El-Khoueiry AB, et al. SWOG S0809: A phase II intergroup trial of adjuvant capecitabine and gemcitabine followed by radiotherapy and concurrent capecitabine in extrahepatic cholangiocarcinoma and gallbladder carcinoma. Journal of Clinical Oncology. 2015;**33**:2617-2622

[25] Thet Cho M. Adjuvant gemcitabine plus docetaxel followed by 5FU chemoradiation for patients with resected pancreaticobiliary cancers: A single-institution, phase II study. Journal of Clinical Oncology. 2014;**32**(Suppl):e22243

[26] Primrose JN, Fox R, Palmer DH, Prasad R, Mirza D, Anthoney AD. Adjuvant capecitabine for biliary tract cancer: The BILCAP randomized study. Journal of Clinical Oncology. 2017;**15**(Suppl):4006

[27] Glimelius B, Hoffman K, Sjoden PO, Jacobsson G, Sellstrom H, Enander LK, et al. Chemotherapy improves survival and quality of life in advanced pancreatic and biliary cancer. Annals of Oncology. 1996;**7**:593-600

[28] Sharma A, Dwary AD, Mohanti BK, et al. Best supportive care compared with chemotherapy for unresectable gall bladder cancer: A randomized controlled study. Journal of Clinical Oncology. 2010;**28**:4581-4586

[29] Valle J, Wasan H, Palmer DH, et al. Cisplatin plus gemcitabine versus gemcitabine for biliary tract cancer. The New England Journal of Medicine. 2010;**362**:1273-1281

[30] Okusaka T, Nakachi K, Fukutomi A, et al. Gemcitabine alone or in combination with cisplatin in patients with biliary tract cancer: A comparative multicentre study in Japan. British Journal of Cancer. 2010;**103**:469-474

[31] Phelip JM, Vendrely V, Jouve JL, et al. Chimioradiothérapie (CHRT: 5-fluoro-uracile, cisplatine, 50 Gy) versus chimiothérapie GEMOX (gemcitabine, oxaliplatine) pour les cancers localement avancés des voies biliaires (CLAVB): essai randomisé de phase II multicentrique (FFCD9902). JFHOD 2013

Chapter 8

Intraoperative ERCP for Management of Gallbladder and Common Bile Duct Stones

Ahmed Abdelraouf Elgeidie

Abstract

It is not an uncommon scenario to have CBD stones in association with gallbladder stones. There is a general agreement in the surgical society that CBD stones should be removed. The classic option is to do open cholecystectomy and CBD exploration. With the emergence of minimally invasive surgery, namely laparoscopic cholecystectomy and ERCP, the therapist has better option to treat such patients such as preoperative ERCP, postoperative ERCP, and laparoscopic CBD exploration. The latest advance in that field is the use of ERCP at the time of laparoscopic cholecystectomy, i.e. intraoperative ERCP. This chapter with discuss the issue of minimally invasive management of cholecystocholedocholithiasis stressing on intraoperative ERCP.

Keywords: laparoscopic cholecystectomy, ERCP, LCBDE, CBD stones, intraoperative ERCP

1. Introduction

Patients undergoing LC may have concomitant CBD stones in about 15% of cases [1, 2]. These CBD stones may pass spontaneously in about one third of cases [3], but the complications of retained CBD stones are often dangerous. These complications include cholangitis, liver abscess, biliary pancreatitis. Therefore, there is a general agreement among biliary surgeons that CBD stones should be removed once detected even if asymptomatic [1, 4].

The orthodox therapeutic option in this setting is to solve the two problems by removing the gallbladder and at the same time retrieving CBD stones via open surgery. In fact this option is a good option with good outcome. Nevertheless, it may be associated with a considerable morbidity (11–14%) and even mortality (0.6–1%) particularly in elderly patients [5].

Two important revolutions had emerged in the past few decades that changed the face of CBD stone management and gave therapists new safe and minimally invasive options when dealing with such patients. The first one was the development of endoscopic retrograde cholangiopancreatography (ERCP) and the second is laparoscopic cholecystectomy (LC). ERCP has become a widely available and routine procedure, whilst open cholecystectomy has largely been replaced by a laparoscopic approach, which is considered the treatment of choice for gallbladder removal since NIH Consensus on 1993 [6].

Nowadays, not only biliary surgeons and endoscopists but also patients prefer minimally invasive options over old open surgery. This is simply because of the well-known benefits of better cosmesis, less adhesions, less wound complications, less postoperative pain and analgesia, and fast recovery.

2. Minimally invasive option

Minimally invasive options for treatment of gallbladder and concomitant CBD stones may be categorized in two sections; one-stage and two-stage options. In the two-stage option, the two pathologies are treated at timely different occasions. This option includes preoperative ERCP followed by LC and LC followed later on by postoperative ERCP. In the one-stage option, the two pathologies are treated in the same sitting under the same anesthesia, and it includes LC/laparoscopic CBD exploration (LCBDE) and LC/intraoperative ERCP.

2.1 Preoperative ERCP followed by LC

In this two-stage strategy the CBD stones are removed firstly to be followed later on by LC at another stetting. Actually this strategy is the most commonly used treatment policy worldwide [7] as it had been proved to be efficient and safe [8–10].

Despite its advantages it has a myriad of disadvantages. Biliary endoscopists may not find CBD stones at the time of ERCP and this means that you are exposing your patient to unnecessary and at the same time risky maneuver. The reported incidence of false negative preoperative ERCP is about 40–70% which is a high figure [11–13]. Ordering magnetic resonance cholangiopancreatography (MRCP) before preoperative ERCP may increase the sensitivity and specificity of preoperative detection of CBD stones [14, 15] but CBD stones may spontaneously pass before ERCP. More than 50% of patients with CBD stones may have spontaneous passage of the stones [16].

At the time of LC, laparoscopists still could identify CBD stones despite successful pre-LC endoscopic clearance during LC. Pierce and collaborators reported an incidence of 12.9% [17]. These stones may be missed at the time of pre-LC ERCP or new stones that passed from the gallbladder onto the CBD in period between the two procedures.

Preoperative ERCP definitely affects the subsequent surgery. Some authors reported more conversion to open cholecystectomy, longer operating time, higher morbidity, especially postoperative infection, and longer hospital stay [18–20].

Finally, the time delay between preoperative ERCP and LC, may allow some patients to escape LC being satisfied by the results of preoperative ERCP [21–23]. Those escaping patients are subjected to recurrent biliary problems [24, 25].

2.2 Post-LC ERCP

Herein, at the first stage the gallbladder is removed by LC to be followed later on by postoperative ERCP as a second stage. The disadvantage of this strategy is obvious. Failed post-LC ERCP, which may the case in up to 5% of cases, necessitates a third stage for operative removal of CBD stones [26, 27].

2.3 LCBDE

In the surgical literature, LCBDE has been proved to be a safe, efficient and cost-effective minimally invasive option [28, 29]. Many authors reported excellent results for LCBDE with a high stone clearance rates up to 100% associated with a low morbidity and mortality rates [30–32].

Besides being a one-stage procedure, the most important advantage of LCBDE is avoidance of ERCP and ES. ERCP is not a totally benign procedure, it may have a short-term consequences as pancreatitis, bleeding and perforation, medium-term complications as cholangitis and recurrent stone formation, or even long-term problems as bile duct malignancy.

In the light of all these advantage, LCBDE would be expectedly to be the standard option for management of gallstones and concomitant CBD stones. But this is not the case in real surgical life for many reasons. LCBDE needs experience and a long learning curve. This is mainly due to the need for laparoscopic suturing skills that must be mastered by the surgeon for T-tube insertion or even primary CBD closure. In case of large, multiple or impacted stones the procedure may be time consuming and exhausting. Finally, LCBDE required specialized instruments that may be not readily available (such as real-time fluoroscopy) or delicate and nondurable (such as fragile 3-mm choledochoscope).

3. Intraoperative ERCP

The most recent advance in management of patients with CCL is intraoperative ERCP [33–36] that was found by many experts to be safe, efficient and cost-effective one-stage option [11, 32–34, 36–39].

3.1 Advantages

Intraoperative ERCP has many theoretical benefits that makes this option of big value. It is a one-session option with single anesthesia and single hospital stay and this is not only cost-effective but safer and seems likable by patients and surgeons. Intraoperative ERCP avoids opening the CBD for stone removal and thereby avoids laparoscopic suturing which needs some experience. Unlike postoperative ERCP, there is no possibility of failure of stone extraction. Simply if intraoperative ERCP failed, stones are removed under the same anesthesia either by open or laparoscopic CBD exploration depending on facilities and expertise. Another final advantage is the performance of ES at intraoperative ERCP. This definitely facilitates subsequent postoperative ERCP if indicated for retrieval of any retained CBD stones.

Nevertheless, all the above mentioned benefits of intraoperative ERCP did not result in widespread application and adoption of this approach. This is because of organizational problems. It may be difficult to have the immediate availability of ERCPist with all required equipment and facilities in the operating room at the time of cholecystectomy.

3.2 Technique

There are many described techniques for performing Intraoperative ERCP during LC but they all fall in two big categories; standard ERCP during LC and combined laparoendoscopic (rendezvous) technique.

3.2.1 Standard ERCP

The first described one was standard ERCP during LC. During LC intraoperative cholangiography is performed and if yielded positive result, intraoperative ERCP is performed in the operating room. After verification of clearance of CBD, LC was continued [37, 40]. This technique has two main shortcomings; firstly, cannulation of the bile duct in the supine position is definitely more difficult than the standard prone/left lateral position and secondly, the resultant bowel distension from endoscopic manipulation may render subsequent LC more challenging.

A variation of this technique is postponing ERCP till after completion of LC and closure of the ports. This is to avoid the two mentioned problems of supine position and bowel distension making LC more demanding [41]. However, the obvious disadvantage of this approach is the problem of failure.

3.2.2 Rendezvous technique

This technique was first described by Cavina et al. [35]. At laparoscopy the surgeon passes a basket through the opened cystic duct and threaded down to the duodenum. At endoscopy a sphincterotome is passed through the scope biopsy channel. The basket caught the sphincterotome and guides it inside the CBD for sphincterotomy.

A simpler modification of the RV technique was proposed by others and now is considered the gold standard technique of intraoperative ERCP [12, 33, 34]. At laparoscopy a standard ERCP guidewire is passed through the opened cystic duct and threaded into the CBD under fluoroscopic guidance till protruding into the duodenum out of the papilla. At endoscopy a snare or basket is passed and catches the protruding guidewire, which is withdrawn into the biopsy channel of the scope and then a standard sphincterotome is threaded over this guidewire for subsequent sphincterotomy (**Figure 1**).

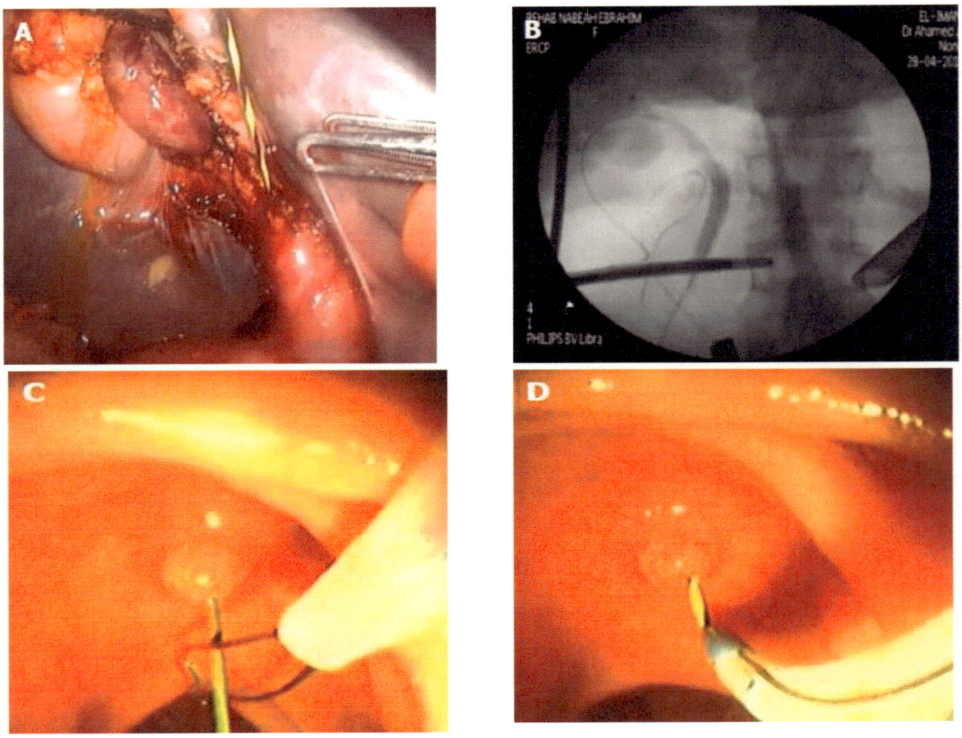

Figure 1.
Rendezvous technique of intraoperative ERCP. (A) Laparoscopic view showing standard ERCP guidewire passing through the cystic duct into CBD; (B) fluoroscopic view showing passage of the guidewire into the duodenum; (C) endoscopic view showing snare catching the protruding guidewire; (D) endoscopic view showing standard sphincterotome threaded over the guidewire for sphincterotomy.

RV technique rapidly became the favorite technique of intraoperative ERCP. This is mainly due to two reasons; the high success cannulation rate in supine position and reduction of postprocedural hyperamylasemia and acute pancreatitis [34, 42, 43]. The obvious cause for reduction of the risk of hyperamylasemia and pancreatitis in intraoperative ERCP compared to standard ERCP is selective cannulation of CBD without inadvertent cannulation and dye injection of pancreatic duct, which is one of the risk factors for post-ERCP pancreatitis [12, 44].

Some technical problems may occur during RV technique. Sometimes it may be difficult for the guidewire to negotiate the spiral valves of the cyst duct. This problem can be overcome by opening the cystic duct as close as possible to its juncture with CBD. Rough manipulation may result in tearing of the cystic duct and this definitely makes subsequent steps more difficult. When there is a deeply impacted stone at the papilla, the guidewire may fail to pass into the duodenum. Finally, bowel distension usually make subsequent LC more difficult. This problem can be easily solved by completely dissecting the Calot triangle before the endoscopic phase [42].

4. Conclusion

Intraoperative ERCP for managing patients with concomitant gallbladder stones and CBD stones is a promising technique that is efficient, cost-effective and safe. The only limitation for its widespread use is lack of immediate availability of endoscopists and endoscopic equipment necessary for the procedure. When local resources and expertise are available it should be offered to fit patients. Surgeons are encouraged to learn ERCP and to use it as an important tool in their hands when dealing with such patients.

Conflict of interest

I have no conflict of interest.

Author details

Ahmed Abdelraouf Elgeidie
Gastrointestinal Surgery Center, Mansoura University, Mansoura, Egypt

*Address all correspondence to: ahmedraoaf8@gmail.com

References

[1] Williams EJ, Green J, Beckingham I, Parks R, Martin D, Lombard M. Guidelines on the management of common bile duct stones (CBDS). Gut. 2008;**57**:1004-1021. DOI: 10.1136/gut.2007.121657

[2] Soltan HM, Kow L, Toouli J. A simple scoring system for predicting bile duct stones in patients with cholelithiasis. Journal of Gastrointestinal Surgery. 2005;**5**:434-437. DOI: 10.1016/S1091-255X(01)80073-1

[3] Collins C, Maguire D, Ireland A, Fitzgerald E, O'Sullivan GC. A prospective study of common bile duct calculi in patients undergoing laparoscopic cholecystectomy: Natural history of choledocholithiasis revisited. Annals of Surgery. 2004;**239**:28-33

[4] Scientific Committee of the European Association for Endoscopic Surgery (E.A.E.S.). Diagnosis and treatment of common bile duct stones (CBDS). Results of a consensus development conference. Surgical Endoscopy. 1998;**12**:856-864. DOI: 10.1007/s004649900729

[5] Phillips EH, Toouli J, Pitt HA, Soper NJ. Treatment of common bile duct stones discovered during cholecystectomy. Journal of Gastrointestinal Surgery. 2008;**12**:624-628. DOI: 10.1007/s11605-007-0452-0

[6] NIH Consensus Development Panel on Gallstones and Laparoscopic Cholecystectomy. Gallstones and laparoscopic cholecystectomy. Surgical Endoscopy. 1993;**7**:271-279. DOI: 10.1007/BF00594118

[7] Freitas ML, Bell RL, Duffy AJ. Choledocholithiasis: Evolving standards for diagnosis and management. World Journal of Gastroenterology. 2006;**12**:3162-3167

[8] Lu J, Xiong XZ, Cheng Y, Lin YX, Zhou RX, You Z, et al. One-stage versus two-stage management for concomitant gallbladder stones and common bile duct stones in patients with obstructive jaundice. The American Surgeon. 2013;**79**:1142-1148

[9] Bansal VK, Misra MC, Rajan K, Kilambi R, Kumar S, Krishna A, et al. Single-stage laparoscopic common bile duct exploration and cholecystectomy versus two-stage endoscopic stone extraction followed by laparoscopic cholecystectomy for patients with concomitant gallbladder stones and common bile duct stones: A randomized controlled trial. Surgical Endoscopy. 2014;**28**:875-885. DOI: 10.1007/s00464-013-3237-4

[10] Li MK, Tang CN, Lai EC. Managing concomitant gallbladder stones and common bile duct stones in the laparoscopic era: A systematic review. Asian Journal of Endoscopic Surgery. 2011;**4**:53-58. DOI: 10.1111/j.1758-5910.2011.00073.x

[11] Erickson RA, Carlson B. The role of endoscopic retrograde cholangiopancreatography in patients with laparoscopic cholecystectomies. Gastroenterology. 1995;**109**:252-263. DOI: 10.1016/0016-5085(95)90292-9

[12] Enochsson L, Lindberg B, Swahn F, Arnelo U. Intraoperative endoscopic retrograde cholangiopancreatography (ERCP) to remove common bile duct stones during routine laparoscopic cholecystectomy does not prolong hospitalization: A 2-year experience. Surgical Endoscopy. 2004;**18**:367-371. DOI: 10.1007/s00464-003-9021-0

[13] Coppola R, Riccioni ME, Ciletti S, Cosentino L, Ripetti V, Magistrelli P, et al. Selective use of endoscopic retrograde cholangiopancreatography to facilitate laparoscopic cholecystectomy

without cholangiography. A review of 1139 consecutive cases. Surgical Endoscopy. 2001;**15**:1213-1216. DOI: 10.1007/s004640080019

[14] Garrow D, Miller S, Sinha D, Conway J, Hoffman BJ, Hawes RH, et al. Endoscopic ultrasound: A meta-analysis of test performance in suspected biliary obstruction. Clinical Gastroenterology and Hepatology. 2007;**5**:616-623. DOI: 10.1016/j.cgh.2007.02.027

[15] Kaltenthaler EC, Walters SJ, Chilcott J, Blakeborough A, Vergel YB, Thomas S. MRCP compared to diagnostic ERCP for diagnosis when biliary obstruction is suspected: A systematic review. BMC Medical Imaging. 2006;**6**:9. DOI: 10.1186/1471-2342-6-9

[16] Lefemine V, Morgan RJ. Spontaneous passage of common bile duct stones in jaundiced patients. Hepatobiliary & Pancreatic Diseases International. 2011;**10**:209-213. DOI: 10.1016/S1499-3872(11)60033-7

[17] Pierce RA, Jonnalagadda S, Spitler JA, Tessier DJ, Liaw JM, Lall SC, et al. Incidence of residual choledocholithiasis detected by intraoperative cholangiography at the time of laparoscopic cholecystectomy in patients having undergone preoperative ERCP. Surgical Endoscopy. 2008;**22**:2365-2372. DOI: 10.1007/s00464-008-9785-3

[18] Ishizaki Y, Miwa K, Yoshimoto J, Sugo H, Kawasaki S. Conversion of elective laparoscopic to open cholecystectomy between 1993 and 2004. The British Journal of Surgery. 2006;**93**:987-991. DOI: 10.1002/bjs.5406

[19] de Vries A, Donkervoort SC, van Geloven AA, Pierik EG. Conversion rate of laparoscopic cholecystectomy after endoscopic retrograde cholangiography in the treatment of choledocholithiasis: Does the time interval matter? Surgical Endoscopy. 2005;**19**:996-1001. DOI: 10.1007/s00464-004-2206-3

[20] Ros A, Gustafsson L, Krook H, Nordgren CE, Thorell A, Wallin G, et al. Laparoscopic cholecystectomy versus mini-laparotomy cholecystectomy: A prospective, randomized, single-blind study. Annals of Surgery. 2001;**234**:741-749. DOI: 10.1097/00000658-200112000-00005

[21] Byrne MF, McLoughlin MT, Mitchell RM, Gerke H, Pappas TN, Branch MS, et al. The fate of patients who undergo "preoperative" ERCP to clear known or suspected bile duct stones. Surgical Endoscopy. 2009;**23**:74-79. DOI: 10.1007/s00464-008-9903-2

[22] Yi SY. Recurrence of biliary symptoms after endoscopic sphincterotomy for choledocholithiasis in patients with gall bladder stones. Journal of Gastroenterology and Hepatology. 2000;**15**:661-664. DOI: 10.1046/j.1440-1746.2000.02192.x

[23] Lau JY, Leow CK, Fung TM, Suen BY, Yu LM, Lai PB, et al. Cholecystectomy or gallbladder in situ after endoscopic sphincterotomy and bile duct stone removal in Chinese patients. Gastroenterology. 2006;**130**:96-103. DOI: 10.1053/j.gastro.2005.10.015

[24] Schiphorst AH, Besselink MG, Boerma D, Timmer R, Wiezer MJ, van Erpecum KJ, et al. Timing of cholecystectomy after endoscopic sphincterotomy for common bile duct stones. Surgical Endoscopy. 2008;**22**:2046-2050. DOI: 10.1007/s00464-008-9764-8

[25] Reinders JS, Goud A, Timmer R, Kruyt PM, Witteman BJ, Smakman N, et al. Early laparoscopic cholecystectomy improves outcomes after endoscopic sphincterotomy for choledochocystolithiasis. Gastroenterology. 2010;**138**:2315-2320. DOI: 10.1053/j.gastro.2010.02.052

[26] Rhodes M, Sussman L, Cohen L, Lewis MP. Randomised trial of laparoscopic exploration of common bile duct versus postoperative endoscopic retrograde cholangiography for common bile duct stones. Lancet. 1998;**351**:159-161. DOI: 10.1016/S0140-6736(97)09175-7

[27] Nathanson LK, O'Rourke NA, Martin IJ, Fielding GA, Cowen AE, Roberts RK, et al. Postoperative ERCP versus laparoscopic choledochotomy for clearance of selected bile duct calculi: A randomized trial. Annals of Surgery. 2005;**242**:188-192. DOI: 10.1097/01.sla.0000171035.57236.d7

[28] Cuschieri A, Croce E, Faggioni A, Jakimowicz J, Lacy A, Lezoche E, et al. EAES ductal stone study. Preliminary findings of multicenter prospective randomized trial comparing two-stage vs single-stage management. Surgical Endoscopy. 1996;**10**:1130-1135. DOI: 10.1007/s004649900264

[29] Tranter SE, Thompson MH. Comparison of endoscopic sphincterotomy and laparoscopic exploration of the common bile duct. The British Journal of Surgery. 2002;**89**:1495-1504. DOI: 10.1046/j.1365-2168.2002.02291.x

[30] Rojas-Ortega S, Arizpe-Bravo D, Marín López ER, CesinSánchez R, Roman GR, Gómez C. Transcystic common bile duct exploration in the management of patients with choledocholithiasis. Journal of Gastrointestinal Surgery. 2003;**7**:492-496. DOI: 10.1016/S1091-255X(03)00026-X

[31] Thompson MH, Tranter SE. All-comers policy for laparoscopic exploration of the common bile duct. The British Journal of Surgery. 2002;**89**:1608-1612. DOI: 10.1046/j.1365-2168.2002.02298.x

[32] Tai CK, Tang CN, Ha JP, Chau CH, Siu WT, Li MK. Laparoscopic exploration of common bile duct in difficult choledo cholithiasis. Surgical Endoscopy. 2004;**18**:910-914. DOI: 10.1007/s00464-003-8216-8

[33] Hong DF, Li JD, Gao M. One hundred and six cases analyses of laparoscopic technique combined with intraoperative cholangiogram and endoscopic sphincterotomy in sequential treatment of cholelithiasis. Chinese Journal of General Surgery. 2003;**15**:648-650

[34] El-Geidie AA. Laparoendoscopic management of concomitant gallbladder stones and common bile duct stones: What is the best technique? Surgical Laparoscopy, Endoscopy & Percutaneous Techniques. 2011;**21**:282-287. DOI: 10.1097/SLE.0b013e3182218908

[35] DePaula AL, Hashiba K, Bafutto M, Zago R, Machado MM. Laparoscopic antegrade sphincterotomy. Surgical Laparoscopy Endoscopy & Percutaneous Techniques. 1993;**3**:157-160

[36] Curet MJ, Pitcher DE, Martin DT, Zucker KA. Laparoscopic antegrade sphincterotomy. A new technique for the management of complex choledocholithiasis. Annals of Surgery. 1995;**221**:149-155. DOI: 10.1097/00000658-199502000-0 0004

[37] Tekin A, Ogetman Z, Altunel E. Laparoendoscopic "rendezvous" versus laparoscopic antegrade sphincterotomy for choledocholithiasis. Surgery. 2008;**144**:442-447. DOI: 10.1016/j.surg.2008.04.013

[38] Ponsky JL, Scheeres DE, Simon I. Endoscopic retrograde cholangioscopy. An adjunct to endoscopic exploration of the common bile duct. The American Surgeon. 1990;**56**:235-237

[39] Fitzgibbons RJ, Deeik RK, Martinez-Serna T. Eight years'

experience with the use of a transcystic common bile duct duodenal double-lumen catheter for the treatment of choledocholithiasis. Surgery. 1998;**124**:699-705; discussion 705-706. DOI: 10.1067/msy.1998.91268

[40] Morino M, Baracchi F, Miglietta C, Furlan N, Ragona R, Garbarini A. Preoperative endoscopic sphincterotomy versus laparoendoscopic rendezvous in patients with gallbladder and bile duct stones. Annals of Surgery. 2006;**244**:889-893; discussion 893-896. DOI: 10.1097/01.sla.0000246913.74870.fc

[41] La Greca G, Barbagallo F, Di Blasi M, Di Stefano M, Castello G, Gagliardo S, et al. Rendezvous technique versus endoscopic retrograde cholangiopancreatography to treat bile duct stones reduces endoscopic time and pancreatic damage. Journal of Laparoendoscopic & Advanced Surgical Techniques. Part A. 2007;**17**:167-171. DOI: 10.1089/lap.2006.0030

[42] Dasari BV, Tan CJ, Gurusamy KS, Martin DJ, Kirk G, McKie L, et al. Surgical versus endoscopic treatment of bile duct stones. Cochrane Database of Systematic Reviews. 2013;**9**:CD003327. DOI: 10.1002/14651858.CD003327

[43] Hong DF, Xin Y, Chen DW. Comparison of laparoscopic cholecystectomy combined with intraoperative endoscopic sphincterotomy and laparoscopic exploration of the common bile duct for cholecystocholedocholithiasis. Surgical Endoscopy. 2006;**20**:424-427

[44] ElGeidie AA, ElShobary MM, Naeem YM. Laparoscopic exploration versus intraoperative endoscopic sphincterotomy for common bile duct stones: A prospective randomized trial. Digestive Surgery. 2011;**28**:424-431. DOI: 10.1159/000331470

Chapter 9

Cystic Artery Variations and Associated Vascular Complications in Laparoscopic Cholecystectomy

Pankaj Prasoon, Tomohiro Katada, Kohei Miura, Yuki Hirose, Jun Sakata and Toshifumi Wakai

Abstract

Substantial knowledge of the arterial supply and its anatomical variations of the gall bladder and liver are important in all the hepatobiliary surgical procedures. The arterial supply of gallbladder called cystic artery (CA) is a vital structure required to get ligated or clipped in the path of laparoscopic cholecystectomy. The possible concerns like intra-operative bleeding or adjoining accidental injuries will almost always be focused on the research consisting of dissection and clipping with cystic artery. Pseudoaneurysm of the cystic artery has additionally been belonging to the presence of acute cholecystitis or pancreatitis. An original supply of CA is usually assessed depending on the existence of hepatic artery variants. Laparoscopic cholecystectomy is really a recent and arduous noninvasive procedure and might even result in substantial unintended effects possibly iatrogenic or in the form of post-procedural complications. The perfect knowledge of anatomy in addition to feasible variation of cystic artery is mandatory. An efficient operative strategy and consciousness are probably the key components with all the results and marginal likelihood of complications, which often can be ultimately attainable. Within this chapter, we have attempted to explore some variations of cystic artery, complications and management.

Keywords: cystic artery (CA), laparoscopic cholecystectomy (LC), proper hepatic artery (PHA), right hepatic artery (RHA), inferior mesenteric artery (IMA)

1. Introduction

Laparoscopic cholecystectomy (LC) is commonly used nowadays to treat numerous conditions and diseases of the gallbladder and biliary tree. It is mandatory to specialists to get acquainted with all the technique, but additionally with anatomical variants of vascular supply in the extrahepatic biliary structures [1]. The cystic artery is often a solitary blood vessel that arises from the right branch from the proper hepatic artery (PHA). It constantly goes to the hepatobiliary triangle, which is encircled superiorly with the inferior surface of the liver, inferiorly with the cystic duct and, the common hepatic duct corresponds to medially [2]. According to Calot's triangle illustration, the superior border is made with the cystic artery [2]. While getting closer to the gallbladder, the cystic artery divides into two branches superficially and deeply running on the anterior and posterior components of the gallbladder, correspondingly. Variants at the originations and course of CA are extremely typical. Uncontrolled arterial bleeding during LC is often a significant issue and might increase the likelihood of biliary duct injury. Consequently, appropriate recognition of the anatomy of the CA is essential. Cystic artery is excessively acknowledged to possess a highly diverse branching pattern. Therefore, given that LC had become the defacto standard to treat cholelithiasis, comprehension of anatomical vascular variations in hepatobiliary surgery has attained significance [3].

2. Types of cystic artery and its variation

2.1 Single cystic artery

The cystic artery commences within the Calot's triangle and most often starting from the right hepatic artery. When getting close to the gallbladder, it bifurcates into deep and superficial branches to the gallbladder neck. The exterior branch proceeds eventually left facet of the gallbladder. The deep branch goes throughout the connective tissues between gallbladder and liver parenchyma. The deep branch engenders really small offshoots to furnish the gallbladder, which anastomoses with all the superficial branches [4]. During open cholecystectomy, such type of CA is laterally located through the cystic duct within Calot's triangle. However in LC procedure, it is merely at the back and a bit much deeper contrary to cystic duct [4]. In a study, such type of variations were documented (73.3%) in 440 of 600 patients [4]. The intricate anatomical deviation among cystic arteries might increase the likelihood of injury throughout LC procedure [5]. Yet in another research, CT images had been analyzed prior to LC, were compared with intra-operative findings and postoperative results. It was witnessed that, cystic artery originating from the right hepatic artery were (76%) in most of the cases, while 55 (60%), CA originating from the right hepatic artery and it undergoes the Calot's triangle and reached the neck of the gallbladder in total of the 91 cases [5]. A single artery to cystic duct together with the conventional configuration of "H shaped" was revealed in 161 (91.47%) patients [6]. Within a current overview of 9800 patients, It is documented that the typical origination of cystic artery were from the RHA (79.02%), where as in 5427 patients (81.5%), origination was found in the hepatobiliary triangle [7]. Variations within cystic artery possessing clinical significance, located anterior to the common hepatic duct in 485 of 2704 patients (17.9%); whereas in 228 (5.4%), out of 4202 patients, located anterior to CBD, correspondingly [7]. A single CA was witnessed in 340 cases out of 740 patients. [8]. Single CA is present in 85% of sufferers out of 300 cases of LC [9]. On standard cholecystectomy, single CA sometimes appears within the hepatobiliary triangle and much more laterally positioned with the cystic duct, although while in laparoscopic view, it could be observed behind and marginally deeper compared to cystic duct [10]. In a recent study by Yang et al., the original source and variety of cystic arteries as well as their relationship together with the Calot's triangle was assessed by CT images and further it was compared with laparoscopic cholecystectomy results. They witnessed single CA was in 53 (73%) of the 73 patients [5]. In one study, normal origin of CA originating from the right hepatic artery was noticed in 72% of patients [11]. In accordance to the reported results, the conventional position of the cystic artery can be found in 70–80% of scenarios [4, 10–12] (**Figure 1A**). Within the study with Kenyan's populations, it had been stated that the CA stood a typical origin from the right hepatic artery in 92.2% of cases, although only one CA supplied the gallbladder within a comparable ratio [13]. With the laparoscopic point of view, a single or a

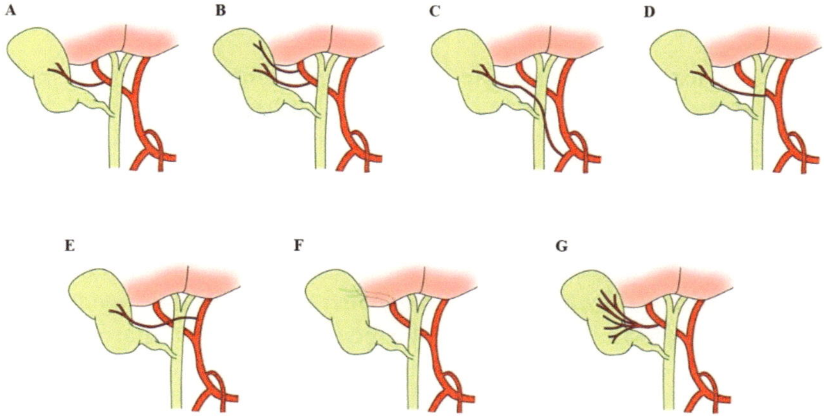

Figure 1.
Schematic illustrations of various anatomic anomalies of cystic artery during LC. (A) Cystic artery origination from right hepatic artery; (B) double cystic artery origination from right hepatic artery; (C) cystic artery origination from gastroduodenal artery; (D) cystic artery origination from aberrant right hepatic artery; (E) cystic artery origination from left hepatic artery; (F) cystic artery origination from liver parenchyma; (G) cystic artery syndrome.

bit larger CA in length necessitates gentle exploration, as it can really be an aberrant hepatic artery, which needs to be dissociated from the cystic duct or gallbladder by cautious dissection [10].

2.2 Double cystic artery

The double cystic artery shows scenarios in which the superficial and deep branches of the CA have independent origins [14] (**Figure 1B**). Double cystic artery could be divided up based upon the position with regards to the bile ducts and portal vein and the hepatobiliary triangle [1, 4, 10]. Concerning the origins of double cystic arteries, they sometimes seem to be with the right hepatic artery or its partitions [1, 15]. According to Loukas et al., double cystic arteries originating both from Right hepatic artery and the posterior superior pancreaticoduodenal artery coexists having an accessory left hepatic artery originating from the left gastric artery [16].

Ding et al.; defined a terminology called "compound cystic artery," in which the cystic arteries endured not just in the hepatobiliary triangle, but additionally outside of it [4]. Congenital absence of the deep branch of CA indicates the presence of an additional CA, and that is often recognized by subsequent hemostasis following LC. The posterior CA is extremely fragile in some instances, and it is frequently cut by electrocoagulation while in dissection. According to one study, such types of likelihood of vessel occurrence in 73 patients (12.2%); i.e. (double cystic artery) right after LC [4]. Suzuki et al. revealed incidence of double cystic artery in 27 cases (11.1%) out from 244 Japanese patients who undergone LC [1]. Zubair et al. noted the most typical variant with double CA in the Pakistani patients during the LC procedure. He witnessed the CA passing over the Calot's triangle, which had been observed in 26 (11.8%) scenarios out of 220 [17]. While in another research double cystic artery was present in only 3 of 300 cases (1%) [9]. In Western communities of Slovenians and Croatians, double cystic artery was documented in 13.6 and 5.5% of cases, correspondingly [10, 15]. In the recent research conducted by Yang et al., all patients experienced LC following the CT examinations [5]. The relationship between CA as well as the Calot's triangle was compared by the interventional radiologist and surgeon. Double cystic arteries were witnessed in 20 (27%) patients [5].

2.3 Cystic artery origination from gastroduodenal artery (GDA)

On few occasions, the CA emanate from the gastroduodenal artery or its branches, it is termed as "a low-lying cystic artery." Its terminal segment getting close to the gallbladder is essential for laparoscopic visual image [10]. On standing point of laparoscopic view, it is actually identified much more superficially or anteriorly to the cystic duct. Therefore, to be the first structure stumbled upon on cholecystectomy. In this instance, there is a probability of its intersection on dissecting the peritoneal replication hooking up the hepatoduodenal ligament to Hartman's pouch with the gall bladder or even the cystic duct. This anatomic deviation was discovered in 9 (4.5%) individuals [10]. The incidence with this anatomic discrepancy varies from 1 to 30% [2, 10, 18].(**Figure 1C**). In a latest review, based on clinically important anatomical variations of the cystic artery, it was witnessed that the aberrant gastroduodenal origination of cystic artery was (1.94%) out of 6898 cases [7]. Ding et al., founded such anatomic variation in 45 patients (7.5%) out from 600 sufferers addressed with LC [4]. As a whole of these terminal branches of artery, the way it approaches the gallbladder is essential for laparoscopic surgeons [4]. Given that, it should not merely be altered at an initial course. However, it is also vulnerable to injuries and hemorrhage throughout the dissection, especially while dealing with peritoneal folds at the joining point of hepatoduodenal ligament to Hartman's pouch on the gallbladder or the cystic duct [4].

2.4 Aberrant right hepatic artery (RHA)

The right hepatic artery (RHA) typically yields several tiny divisions providing gallbladder in contrast to a solitary cystic artery (**Figure 1D**). When masked by the gallbladder in the gallbladder fossa, it is prone to get the injury by cautery directly or by thermal injuries [10]. With the laparoscopic standpoint, a single large cystic artery necessitates gentle exploration, as it might be an aberrant hepatic artery, which needs to be dissociated with the cystic duct or gallbladder which additionally needs meticulous exploration [10]. The biliary anatomy of the Calot's triangle and extrahepatic vascular supply is widely known to become unpredictable and extremely diverse [19]. This allows a persistent obstacle to the surgeon carrying out LC. Cautious dissection of the cystic duct and artery is needed having consistent thoughts within the several anatomical chances to stay clear of either conversion necessitating postoperative bleeding or biliary leak. A replaced RHA is observed in 15–25% of patients, that the great majority disclose the RHA branching from the superior mesenteric artery [20, 21]. Inadvertent RHA ligation in cholecystectomy has become linked to liver ischemia, occasionally warranting resection of affected lobes of liver [22]. An aberrant RHA adherent to the cystic duct and gallbladder neck is referred to one of the most uncommon defects [19, 23]. Anatomical variants are frequent; in 6–16%, the right hepatic artery flows intently parallel to the cystic duct and could be mistakenly ligated during the LC, the structures within the triangle of Calot's are usually not evidently recognized [24]. Andall et al.; noted aberrant RHA origination of (5.58%), 385 out from 6898 cases. An aberrant RHA originating from the celiac trunk is an extremely unusual anatomical variant. Nevertheless, it might be connected with an irregular path of the cystic artery. Specialists have to know anatomical variations of the extrahepatic biliary tree and arterial supply in order to avoid feasible injuries throughout LC [25]. According to recent publicized research, focusing on the patients with combined bile duct and hepatic artery injuries during LC revealed, formation of liver abscesses in three of four cases and stricture's anastomotic site by 50% of four sufferers; on the other hand, these complications just weren't recognized in cases with separated biliary duct injuries [26].

The earlier LC studies demonstrated an anomaly of right hepatic artery and were being disrupted during excessive hemorrhage throughout Calot's triangle dissection [27]. The outline with the surgery described the explanation for blood loss and also the intra-operative management with unspecified amounts of clips [27]. Ding et al., witnessed aberrant RHA in 18 (3%) of cases in their study [4]. The complicated structure of hepatic artery tends to make the hilar and perihilar area much more hazardous and vulnerable to a variety of traumas. The potential for biliary injuries might be of interest in patients who endure complicated or extended dissection with the Calot's triangle, accompanied by the roll-out of discomfort, fever and altered liver function assessments [28].

2.5 Aberrant left hepatic artery

The cystic artery in some instances emanates from the left hepatic artery, heading for the tunnel or through the liver and attaining the center of the gallbladder body or within the gall bladder fossa where it bifurcates it into two branches, which are namely called ascending and descending branches [10] (**Figure 1E**). This CA variance is simply not observed on endoscopic visualization with the hepatobiliary triangle, consequently necessitating extreme caution when treatment of gall bladder with the fossa [10]. Within one study, this sort of CA variation with typical caliber was discovered in 2 (1%) patients [10]. In accordance with the literature, it possesses an occurrence of 4%, where it was acknowledged and clipped [29]. The findings of CA origin were being with the left hepatic artery (2.07%), 143 out from 6898 cases. An aberrant RHA originating from the celiac trunk is an extremely uncommon anatomical variant. Nevertheless, it could be connected with an irregular path of the CA. Specialists should always keep in mind about the extrahepatic biliary tree and arterial supply anatomical variations to counteract attainable injuries while performing LC [25].

2.6 Cystic artery origination from liver parenchyma

As outlined by Ding et al. [4]; This CA pierces the hepatic parenchyma getting close to the gallbladder base (**Figure 1F**). It usually situates inside the right lateral to the edge of gallbladder body and bottom part. Even so, a few are found in the middle of the gallbladder bed or located left lateral of gallbladder base. Hardly any other arterial blood vessels are located inside Calot's triangle [4]. This anatomic variation with the cystic artery is just not witnessed right until hemorrhaging and is because of dissection of the gallbladder fundus. It is sometimes complicated to understand more about and needs cautious dissection. It was witnessed in 15 patients (2.5%) within one another study [4].

2.7 Cystic artery syndrome

Suzuki et al.; referred to a condition known as "cystic artery syndrome", in which the CA originates from the right hepatic artery, but uncommonly has a course that wraps across the cystic duct [1] (**Figure 1G**). They suggested that this course could result in reduced blood flow in the cystic duct, which exhibits clinically within the patient as cholelithiasis [1]. According to Zubair et al., this syndrome was discovered within 2% of the patients who underwent LC procedure [17].

2.8 Abnormal origination of cystic artery

Andall et al. lately have summarized the experiences of 55 experts, they analyzed 9800 cases and discovered only 20 instances where the CA arise straight from the superior mesentric artery (SMA) [7]. An uncommon scenario has been documented possessing CA arising from the SMA with abnormal branching in the CT and MRI within a Japanese woman cadaver [30]. The CA typically come across the ventral facet with the portal vein as well as the posterior side of the common bile duct. Additionally, in their case the CA have origination with the SMA and RHA and they leaped concurrent to Calot's triangle [30]. Consequently, in such instances, it is sometimes complicated for medical professionals to evaluate the origination of CA on account of the SMA [30]. The absence of congenital cystic artery was documented in 33 of 9836 (0.34%) cases [7]. While in another study, scholars mentioned the advantages of computed tomography angiography (CTA), and estimated that, it is quicker, much less intrusive and is through with considerably fewer irradiation exposure. CTA offers an appropriate and efficient depiction of cystic artery vessels in 924% of cases (95% CI, 87–98%) [7]. Nonetheless, variations, for instance, small or short CA, origins from aberrant hepatic artery or from an additional vessel completely results in the CA not passing throughout the cystohepatic triangle [7].

3. Complications associated with cystic artery injuries

3.1 Twisted cystic artery

The signs and symptoms of torsion imitate acute cholecystitis, but various clinical attributes (slim person, older people, and spine problems) and image conclusions are helpful for differentiating it from standard acute cholecystitis [31]. Even so, preoperative recognition continues to be challenging to identify the anomalies of vessels. Considering torsion of CA, it was initially reported in 1898. There are almost 500 cases have been acknowledged inside the literary works, and many of them were diagnosed throughout the surgical procedure [32]. The ultrasonography, computed tomography (CT), and magnetic resonance imaging (MRI) have already been stated to be helpful for proper diagnosis of gallbladder torsion such as twisting of the pedicle of the cystic duct and gallbladder mesentery designated as "whirl sign" [33]. Variety of twisted CA by 3D CT, angiography signifies unique and primary verification with this concern that enables definitive medical diagnosis and obviates the entire overall performance of other assessments [32]. Whenever a patient is assumed of owning torsion with the gallbladder, 3D-CT angiography ought to be carried out for making an earlier significant and exact diagnosis [32].

3.2 Cystic artery pseudoaneurysm (CAP)

Pseudoaneurysm of the cystic artery is actually an uncommon side-effect right after laparoscopic cholecystectomy (**Figure 2**). CA involvement is documented significantly less in the literature. Pseudoaneurysm formation is resulted in by vascular injuries. The important causes consist of arterial access procedures, accident trauma, and surgical trauma [34]. Cystic artery pseudoaneurysm which develops carrying out a cholecystectomy and leading to upper gastrointestinal bleeding are usually an unusual entity, with merely four instances referred to inside the literature [35] .Generally, in most patients (80%), the PSA typically presents roughly a month following LC surgery; on the other hand, delayed PSA presentation after 5 years following the surgical procedure had been documented in the literature [36, 37].

Emergency abdominal angiogram unveiled a CA stump pseudoaneurysm, without any proof of active contrast extravasation and it was managed by coiling

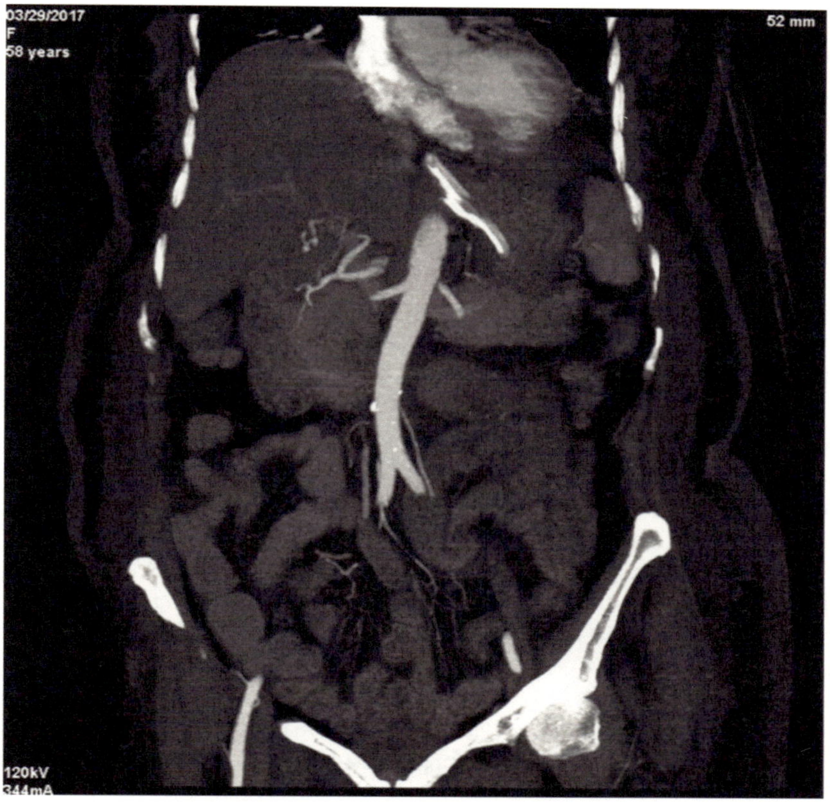

Figure 2.
Pseudoaneurysm in the hepatic artery after radical cholecystectomy.

or embolization's technique, consequently the patient did not have any additional hemorrhagic episodes. In cases like this, an angiogram and embolization in contrast to surgical treatment are the most preferred method of management equally when

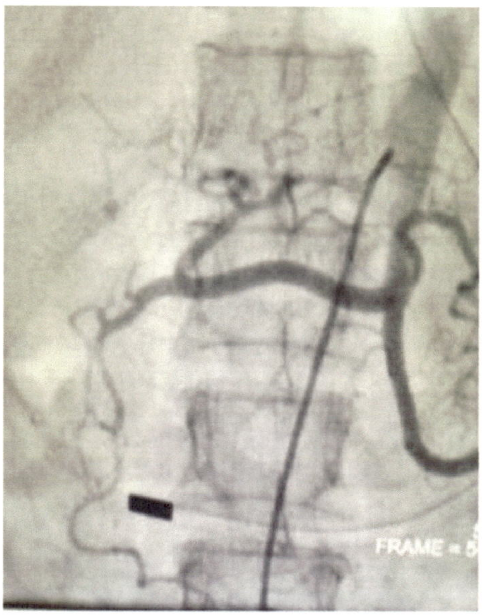

Figure 3.
After the post-embolization of the pseudo aneurysm.

it comes to treatment and diagnosis (**Figure 3**). The existence of a dilated cystic artery stump on angiogram adhering to cholecystectomy is definitely the threatening indicator even without the active extravasation of contrast [35]. The signs and symptoms might appear during the early postoperative period or as late as 4 months following surgical procedure. One of the several attainable causes includes the unnecessary use of electrocautery throughout the dissection at the infundibulum of the gallbladder, leading to thermal damage to the vascular wall, and break down in the inner wall of the cystic artery. A result of exposure to the tip of the metal clip utilized to occlude the cystic duct [38]. The management of their patient incorporated several plans such as attaining hemostasis, managing the cystic duct stump leak, alleviating obstructive jaundice, managing the infections with antibiotics, and depleting the intra-abdominal collection [34].

3.3 Hemobilia due to cystic artery pseudoaneurysm

The mixed injuries of bile ducts and vessels create the pathologic vascular-biliary interconnection and also the hemorrhage with the bile duct, which can be described as hemobilia [39]. Therefore, hemobilia has turned into a specific issue in the laparoscopic age. The likelihood of hemobilia right after an emergency LC for acute cholecystitis (within just 72 h) had been stated to be 0.001%, although it is been witnessed being 0.0003% for all those going through an elective LC [40]. Bile acids are potent solubilizers of lipid membrane for their cytotoxic and amphipathic qualities, leading to cell death in patients with bile leaks; it has been postulated to result in immediate deterioration and break down in the vascular walls, ultimately causing a PSA [41, 42]. Hemobilia has been considered to be the most prevalent presentation (90%), although abdominal pain (70%) and jaundices (60%) are also typical presentations [40, 43]. CAP is usually an unusual entity and therefore, there is absolutely no comprehensive agreement to the medical treatments for this problem. The potential risk of a PSA rupture relates to its dimensions, having a greater than 10 times risk in the event the aneurysm is much larger than 5 cm [44]. A hold off in presentation after thermal injuries could possibly be as a result of charring of the vessel which may get separate several days or weeks later, especially in the existence of bile [40]. The pathophysiology of aneurysmal dilatation of the cystic artery in the existence of calculus cholecystitis just isn't apparent. However, it is considered that the artery is eroded possibly by immediate tension of gallstones or swelling from the arterial wall [45]. This subsequently contributes to harm the adventitia with the localized weak point within the vessel wall and development of the pseudoaneurysm [45].

Hemobilia induced by non-iatrogenic injuries of the CA is really an intense uncommon but attainable etiology, and thus it has to be deemed. Pseudoaneurysm in the CA is an extremely unusual reason behind hemobilia, and its particular pathogenesis remains to be ambiguous [46]. Cholecystitis could produce arterial wall weakness and necrosis leading hemobilia [46]. Many experts have revealed that bleeding pseudoaneurysm of the cystic artery as a result of re-activation of the continual cholecystitis treated by endovascular embolization and subsequent cholecystectomy [47]. Whenever a sufferer presents with significant gastrointestinal internal bleeding, an ascending total bilirubin level and recent hepatobiliary treatment or intervention, a higher index of suspicions is definitely required [48]. Loizides et al.; evaluated altogether, 25 reported cases since 1983–2015 and found that pseudoaneurysm of CA is to be secondary to acute and chronic cholecystitis [45]. During its natural course, a PSA will steadily develop in its dimensions prior to rupture, seen in 21–80% of cases [49]. The rupture of a PSA in the peritoneal cavity may be possibly usual to hypovolemic shock or might be comprised quickly with the encompassing tissue also known as "double rupture phenomenon," since the preliminary comprised hemorrhage might be accompanied by additional blood loss, which can be more severe situation [36].

Unattended hemobilia presents an instantaneous risk to life. It can result in acute hemodynamic imbalances, requiring diagnosis, accessibility, and control over the pseudoaneurysm. Arterial-phase CT is an excellent initial noninvasive mode of detection of LC complication's [34]. This technology not only help to gauge intra-abdominal collection, biliary tree dilatation, and doable bile duct injury, but also to visualize pseudoaneurysms or hemorrhage [34] Several different treatment methods have already been documented within the literature together with selective embolization and coiling, open cholecystectomy with ligation of the aneurysm, or perhaps a two-step approach involving radiological treatments for the pseudoaneurysm accompanied by an elective cholecystectomy [45]. Angiography is a significant restorative technique simply because it make possible for embolization of the cystic pseudoaneurysm, transforming an urgent scenario to a semi elective one [50]. It has a substantial proportion of good results attaining hemostasis in 75–100% of sufferers with hemobilia [50], with a reported of less than 2% [51].

Some patients having typical obstructive jaundice and hemophilia may additionally need endoscopic retrograde cholangiopancreatography, CBD exploration or transhepatic biliary drainage to vacate the clot in the event the jaundice doesn't get relieved [49, 52]. Natural or spontaneous rupture of normal cystic artery is undoubtedly an extremely exceptional reason behind hemoperitoneum [53]. Medical co-morbidity, for instance, arteriosclerosis, diabetes, arterial hypertension and long-term usage of corticosteroid are the most prevalent components liable for vascular fragility [53]. Selective embolization is an efficient and also a noninvasive treatment alternative, which can result in ischemic gallbladder necrosis few days following the treatment [53]. The patients having good hemodynamically status, cholecystectomy can be carried out averting biliary ischemic problems and also the related morbidity and mortality [53].

3.4 Hematemesis due to cystic artery pseudoaneurysm (CAP)

Dependent upon the latency from surgery to presentation, the rate of bleeding differs from the minimum to enormous, with the increased amount of blood loss are much more likely in later presentations [39]. Some possible components of injury considered to play a role in CAP incorporate the unnecessary use of electrocautery when taking apart the infundibulum from the gallbladder, which might trigger thermal damage to the vascular wall and erosion of the tip of the metal clip utilized to ligate the cystic duct into the internal walls of the cystic artery [38]. In cases with repeated hematemesis and a medical history of earlier biliary interventions, upper endoscopy is undoubtedly a suitable first diagnostic step. Direct visualization of blood emanating from the ampulla of vater, diagnostic of hemobilia, is hardly ever experienced [54]. If recurring endoscopic and cholangiographic assessments are not able to uncover a possible bleeding point, angiography may be recommended as the next phase in assessment [54]. Surgical ligation via an open or laparoscopic approach is recognized as second-line treatments for pseudoaneurysm of hepatic artery and CAP, restricted to controls exactly where an angiographic approach isn't feasible or does not work out [54]. In another study, they assessed the importance of choledochoscopy within the evaluation of hemobilia, considering that several EGDs and ERCPs skipped diagnosing, contrary to choledochoscopic visual image of the clip, eroding into the cystic duct remnant by having an adjoining soft-tissue protuberance was the initial indication of potential vascular injury, resulting in the right examination and remedial assistance [55]. Gallbladder ischemia is an issue for patients having an intact gallbladder that endure embolization of the cystic artery. Therefore, in such circumstances gall bladder removal is normally carried out right after embolization procedure [56].

CAPs are unusual but possibly despondent complications of LC procedures. Right upper quadrant pain, hemorrhaging, and jaundice after biliary intervention are an indication of hemobilia, a typical manifestation of pseudoaneurysm, even though introductory signs and symptoms can differ considerably. In the cases where the PSA continues to grow following preliminary management with TAE, following operative management had been documented through which an exploratory laparotomy and ligation of the nourishing vessel ended in an entire recuperation [57]. Infection might also result in a high-risk of vascular suture rupture right after ligation of the artery; within this report, the patient passed away 2 days following surgical repair of a PSA as a result of severe bleeding from GI tract [58]. Gastrointestinal internal bleeding may perhaps present as hematemesis or melena, depending on the rate of blood loss [59]. Erosion on the PSA in GI tract or into the cystic duct stump or forming a fistula between these two structures was earlier documented [58, 60–62]. An increased index chart of diagnostic doubts is really important for earlier acknowledgement and treating this additional unwanted effect. In combination with endoscopy, cholangiography, angiography, and choledochoscopy might be helpful diagnostic resources in order to evaluate of suspected hemobilia [55]. Lately, numerous scientific studies have documented the effective treatments for PSAs by injecting thrombin straight into the hepatic artery aneurysm [37, 63].

On the other hand, embolization employing this approach could possibly be not discerning. It could result in unwanted additional complications, for instance, infarctions of liver and bowel; adding small quantities of thrombin with real-time sonography and Doppler assistance may perhaps lessen this threat [37]. Alternatively, angiographic embolization might be related to considerable hazards, such as shatter in the PSA throughout coil's embolization, an expansion in the thrombosis within the RHA, necrosis, hemorrhage, abscess creation and CBD stricture resulting from poor vascular supply [64–66]. A current review discovered that post-embolization syndrome took place in 9 out from 14 sufferers, and it was linked to the ages of the patient as well as time period relating to the LC procedure and TAE therapy [67]. Some others have recommended usage of a protected stent when dealing with the PSA to be able to sustain blood circulation towards liver preventing additional complications relevant to diminished circulation [68]. Stents could also be used for individuals with accompanying hepatic artery stenosis and PSAs [68]. From a technical perspective, the positioning of the stent for the PSA in the RHA is recognized as complicated owing its far away position, more compact dimension and quite often intricate or transformed [68]. In one report, a patient presented with acute pancreatitis due to corrosion of TAE coils in the CBD subsequently 24 months after the LC [69].

Nevertheless, as a result of substantial advancements in catheter-based treatment plans now are generally given TAE by occluding the providing vascular supply with various embolic agents, which includes gel foam, coils, N-butyl cyanoacrylate and thrombin, ahead of preferably embolizing the vessel proximal and distal towards the PSA to avoid equity filling up in the PSA [37, 60, 65, 66, 70, 71]. In 82% of scenarios, embolization was documented typically effective while, surgical procedures needed in remainder 18% of the subjects [36]. When coils are utilized, they are able to the originator of thrombosis; consequently, in sufferers with considerable coagulopathies, the blood vessel might still continue to be distinct regardless of embolization plus the course of action could possibly be inadequate to managing blood loss [72]. In modest PSAs, glue works extremely well as an alternative because the adhesive contours towards the type of PSA [73]. Additionally, coil's positioning could be tricky in individuals having a modest PSA [71]. In some instances, equally techniques could be implemented [71].

Failing to excise the PSA may bring about its burst since the aneurysm is usually inflamed and infected. An infection may also result in a high-risk of vascular suture split adhering to ligation of the artery; within a review, a person passed away 2 days following surgical repair of a PSA due to catastrophic gastrointestinal hemorrhage [58]. In the event wherein the PSA continues to be expanded following preliminary management with TAE, following operative management had been documented by which an exploratory laparotomy and ligation of the nourishing vessel ended in an entire recuperation [57]. Excision helps to ensure that a PSA won't expand resulting from continual arterial blood pressure; furthermore, failing to excise the PSA may bring about its burst because the aneurysm is frequently contaminated [72]. A number of people who typical to hemobilia and obstructive jaundice may additionally need endoscopic retrograde cholangiopancreatography and transhepatic biliary drainage while in some circumstances CBD exploration to vacate the blood clot in the event the jaundice won't get better [49, 52]. Operative control over to substantial hemobilia is apparently effective for 90% of patients, with rebleeding and fatality rates of lower than 5 and 10%, correspondingly [66].

4. Summary

Most often, vascular injuries and biliary duct injuries may occur concomitantly during the LC procedure. They arise more frequently than contemplated formerly, and it is witnessed much more proximal in LC contrast to those observed in open surgical procedure. Ultimately, it enhances the fatality rate. However, it could potentially cause greater morbidity and endanger the long-term functional outcomes of biliary reconstruction by triggering anastomotic strictures. When recognized earlier, there is certainly some space for restoration and reconstruction, even though this is contentious. Where as in delayed instances, it appears to be acceptable not to consider the vascular injuries by itself.

A hepatic or cystic artery PSA following the LC procedure is definitely infrequent. However, when it ensues occurs as life-threatening complications. The delayed presentation of the situation, which could take place weeks following the surgical procedure, and the typical symptoms with gastrointestinal internal bleeding can potentially lead to incorrect diagnosis or late treatment. Consequently, a higher index of clinical suspicions is needed for patients with inexplicable GI hemorrhage after having the LC procedure. A contrast CT scan or angiogram typically verifies the diagnosing, and trans arterial embolization is most likely the defacto standard of management, having a higher rate of success. On the other hand, operative treatment is essential for cases where TAE is unachievable or does not work out. Safety measures ought to be taken to prevent vascular injury while conducting the LC in order to prevent a PSA, especially when the cholecystectomy procedure is essentially problematic. An increased likelihood of symptomatic suspicion is needed for earlier recognition and management of this unwanted effect. In combination with endoscopy, cholangiography, angiography, and choledochoscopy could be efficient diagnostic tools while in the evaluation of assumed hemobilia. Specialist's consultation is mandatory while having any diagnostic and operative dilemma during the LC procedure in order to deter the unwanted complications and to attain the optimal consequences.

Author details

Pankaj Prasoon, Tomohiro Katada, Kohei Miura, Yuki Hirose, Jun Sakata and Toshifumi Wakai*

Division of Digestive and General Surgery, Niigata University Graduate School of Medical and Dental Sciences, Niigata, Japan

*Address all correspondence to: wakait@med.niigata-u.ac.jp

References

[1] Suzuki M, Akaishi S, Rikiyama T, Naitoh T, Rahman MM, Matsuno S. Laparoscopic cholecystectomy, Calot's triangle, and variations in cystic arterial supply. Surgical Endoscopy. 2000;**14**(2):141-144

[2] Chen TH, Shyu JF, Chen CH, Ma KH, Wu CW, Lui WY, et al. Variations of the cystic artery in Chinese adults. Surgical Laparoscopy, Endoscopy & Percutaneous Techniques. 2000;**10**(3):154-157

[3] Polguj M, Podgorski M, Hogendorf P, Topol M. Variations of the hepatobiliary vasculature including coexistence of accessory right hepatic artery with unusually arising double cystic arteries: Case report and literature review. Anatomical Science International. 2014;**89**(3):195-198

[4] Ding YM, Wang B, Wang WX, Wang P, Yan JS. New classification of the anatomic variations of cystic artery during laparoscopic cholecystectomy. World Journal of Gastroenterology. 2007;**13**(42):5629-5634

[5] Xia J, Zhang Z, He Y, Qu J, Yang J. Assessment and classification of cystic arteries with 64-detector row computed tomography before laparoscopic cholecystectomy. Surgical and Radiologic Anatomy. 2015;**37**(9):1027-1034

[6] Rashid A, Mushtaque M, Bali RS, Nazir S, Khuroo S, Ishaq S. Artery to cystic duct: A consistent branch of cystic artery seen in laparoscopic cholecystectomy. Anatomy Research International. 2015;**2015**:847812

[7] Andall RG, Matusz P, du Plessis M, Ward R, Tubbs RS, Loukas M. The clinical anatomy of cystic artery variations: A review of over 9800 cases. Surgical and Radiologic Anatomy. 2016;**38**(5):529-539

[8] Singh K, Singh R, Kaur M. Clinical reappraisal of vasculobiliary anatomy relevant to laparoscopic cholecystectomy. Journal of Minimal Access Surgery. 2017;**13**(4):273-279

[9] Talpur KA, Laghari AA, Yousfani SA, Malik AM, Memon AI, Khan SA. Anatomical variations and congenital anomalies of extra hepatic biliary system encountered during laparoscopic cholecystectomy. The Journal of the Pakistan Medical Association. 2010;**60**(2):89-93

[10] Balija M, Huis M, Nikolic V, Stulhofer M. Laparoscopic visualization of the cystic artery anatomy. World Journal of Surgery. 1999;**23**(7):703-707. discussion 7

[11] Hugh TB, Kelly MD, Li B. Laparoscopic anatomy of the cystic artery. American Journal of Surgery. 1992;**163**(6):593-595

[12] Daseler EH, Anson BJ, et al. The cystic artery and constituents of the hepatic pedicle; a study of 500 specimens. Surgery, Gynecology & Obstetrics. 1947;**85**(1):47-63

[13] Saidi H, Karanja TM, Ogengo JA. Variant anatomy of the cystic artery in adult Kenyans. Clinical Anatomy (New York, NY). 2007;**20**(8):943-945

[14] Michels NA. Newer anatomy of the liver and its variant blood supply and collateral circulation. American Journal of Surgery. 1966;**112**(3):337-347

[15] Mlakar B, Gadzijev EM, Ravnik D, Hribernik M. Anatomical variations of the cystic artery. European Journal of Morphology. 2003;**41**(1):31-34

[16] Loukas M, Fergurson A, Louis RG, Colborn GL. Multiple variations of the hepatobiliary vasculature including double cystic arteries, accessory left

hepatic artery and hepatosplenic trunk: A case report. Surgical and Radiologic Anatomy. 2006;**28**(5):525-528

[17] Zubair M, Habib L, Mirza RM, Cnanna MA, Yousuf M, Quraishy MS. Anatomical variations of cystic artery: Telescopic facts. The Medical Journal of Malaysia. 2012;**67**(5):494-496

[18] Sarkar AK, Roy TS. Anatomy of the cystic artery arising from the gastroduodenal artery and its choledochal branch—A case report. Journal of Anatomy. 2000;**197**(Pt 3): 503-506

[19] Blecha MJ, Frank AR, Worley TA, Podbielski FJ. Aberrant right hepatic artery in laparoscopic cholecystectomy. Journal of the Society of Laparoendoscopic Surgeons. 2006;**10**(4):511-513

[20] Jones RM, Hardy KJ. The hepatic artery: A reminder of surgical anatomy. Journal of the Royal College of Surgeons of Edinburgh. 2001;**46**(3):168-170

[21] Hiatt JR, Gabbay J, Busuttil RW. Surgical anatomy of the hepatic arteries in 1000 cases. Annals of Surgery. 1994;**220**(1):50-52

[22] Uenishi T, Hirohashi K, Tanaka H, Fujio N, Kubo S, Kinoshita H. Right hepatic lobectomy for recurrent cholangitis after bile duct and hepatic artery injury during laparoscopic cholecystectomy: Report of a case. Hepato-Gastroenterology. 1999;**46**(28):2296-2298

[23] Covey AM, Brody LA, Maluccio MA, Getrajdman GI, Brown KT. Variant hepatic arterial anatomy revisited: Digital subtraction angiography performed in 600 patients. Radiology. 2002;**224**(2):542-547

[24] Scott-Conner CE, Hall TJ. Variant arterial anatomy in laparoscopic cholecystectomy. American Journal of Surgery. 1992;**163**(6):590-592

[25] Katagiri H, Sakamoto T, Okumura K, Lefor AK, Kubota T. Aberrant right hepatic artery arising from the celiac trunk: A potential pitfall during laparoscopic cholecystectomy. Asian Journal of Endoscopic Surgery. 2016;**9**(1):72-74

[26] Gupta N, Solomon H, Fairchild R, Kaminski DL. Management and outcome of patients with combined bile duct and hepatic artery injuries. Archives of Surgery (Chicago, Ill: 1960). 1998;**133**(2):176-181

[27] Martino V, Ferrarese A, Bindi M, Marola S, Gentile V, Rivelli M, et al. Abnormal right hepatic artery injury resulting in right hepatic atrophy: Diagnosed by laparoscopic cholecystectomy. Open Medicine (Warsaw, Poland). 2015;**10**(1):535-537

[28] Mirza DF, Narsimhan KL, Ferraz Neto BH, Mayer AD, McMaster P, Buckels JA. Bile duct injury following laparoscopic cholecystectomy: Referral pattern and management. The British Journal of Surgery. 1997;**84**(6):786-790

[29] Rocko JM, Di Gioia JM. Calot's triangle revisited. Surgery, Gynecology & Obstetrics. 1981;**153**(3):410-414

[30] Yakura T, Hayashi S, Terayama H, Miyaki T, Nakano T, Naito M. A case of a cystic artery arising from the superior mesenteric artery with abnormal branching of the celiac trunk. BMC Research Notes. 2017;**10**(1):526

[31] Lau WY, Fan ST, Wong SH. Acute torsion of the gall bladder in the aged: A re-emphasis on clinical diagnosis. The Australian and New Zealand Journal of Surgery. 1982;**52**(5):492-494

[32] Yokoi T, Miyata K, Yuasa N, Takeuchi E, Goto Y, Miyake H, et al. Twisted cystic artery disclosed by 3-dimensional computed tomography angiography for torsion of the gallbladder. American Journal of Surgery. 2011;**201**(5):e33-e34

[33] Chou CT, Chen RC, Yang AD, Wu HK. Gallbladder torsion: Preoperative diagnosis by MDCT. Abdominal Imaging. 2007;**32**(5):657-659

[34] To K, Lai EC, Chung DT, Chan OC, Tang CN. Cystic artery pseudoaneurysm with haemobilia after laparoscopic cholecystectomy. Hong Kong Medical Journal [Xianggang yi xue za zhi]. 2018;**24**(2):203-205

[35] Moses V, Keshava SN, Wann VC, Joseph P, Sitaram V. Cystic artery pseudoaneurysm after laparoscopic cholecystectomy presenting as haemobilia: A case report. Tropical Gastroenterology. 2008;**29**(2):107-109

[36] Bulut T, Yamaner S, Bugra D, Akyuz A, Acarli K, Poyanli A. False aneurysm of the hepatic artery after laparoscopic cholecystectomy. Acta Chirurgica Belgica. 2002;**102**(6):459-463

[37] Kumar A, Sheikh A, Partyka L, Contractor S. Cystic artery pseudoaneurysm presenting as a complication of laparoscopic cholecystectomy treated with percutaneous thrombin injection. Clinical Imaging. 2014;**38**(4):522-525

[38] De Molla Neto OL, Ribeiro MA, Saad WA. Pseudoaneurysm of cystic artery after laparoscopic cholecystectomy. HPB: The Official Journal of the International Hepato Pancreato Biliary Association. 2006;**8**(4):318-319

[39] Wen F, Dong Y, Lu ZM, Liu ZY, Li W, Guo QY. Hemobilia after laparoscopic cholecystectomy: Imaging features and management of an unusual complication. Surgical Laparoscopy, Endoscopy & Percutaneous Techniques. 2016;**26**(1):e18-e24

[40] Sansonna F, Boati S, Sguinzi R, Migliorisi C, Pugliese F, Pugliese R. Severe hemobilia from hepatic artery pseudoaneurysm. Case Reports in Gastrointestinal Medicine. 2011;**2011**:925142

[41] Madanur MA, Battula N, Sethi H, Deshpande R, Heaton N, Rela M. Pseudoaneurysm following laparoscopic cholecystectomy. Hepatobiliary & Pancreatic Diseases International. 2007;**6**(3):294-298

[42] Bin Traiki TA, Madkhali AA, Hassanain MM. Hemobilia post laparoscopic cholecystectomy. Journal of Surgical Case Reports. 2015;**2015**(2):rju159

[43] Nicholson T, Travis S, Ettles D, Dyet J, Sedman P, Wedgewood K, et al. Hepatic artery angiography and embolization for hemobilia following laparoscopic cholecystectomy. Cardio Vascular and Interventional Radiology. 1999;**22**(1):20-24

[44] Bulut T, Yamaner S, Bugra D, Akyuz A, Acarli K, Poyanli A. False aneurysm of the hepatic artery after laparoscopic cholecystectomy. Acta Chirurgica Belgica. 2002;**102**(6):459-463

[45] Loizides S, Ali A, Newton R, Singh KK. Laparoscopic management of a cystic artery pseudoaneurysm in a patient with calculus cholecystitis. International Journal of Surgery Case Reports. 2015;**14**:182-185

[46] Liang X, Lu JM, Meng N, Jin RA, Cai XJ. Hemorrhagic shock caused by rupture of cystic artery pseudoaneurysm secondary to calculous cholecystitis. Chinese Medical Journal. 2013;**126**(23):4590-4591

[47] Trombatore C, Scilletta R, Bellavia N, Trombatore P, Magnano SLV, Petrillo G, et al. Acute hemobilia from a pseudoaneurysm of the cystic artery arising from the left hepatic artery: Case report and literature review. International Journal of Surgery Case Reports. 2017;**37**:60-64

[48] Demyttenaere SV, Hassanain M, Halwani Y, Valenti D, Barkun JS. Massive hemobilia. Canadian Journal

of Surgery Journal [Canadien de Chirurgie]. 2009;**52**(4):E109-Ee10

[49] Hadj AK, Goodwin M, Schwalb H, Nikfarjam M. Pseudoaneurysm of the hepatic artery. Journal of Gastrointestinal Surgery: Official Journal of the Society for Surgery of the Alimentary Tract. 2011;**15**(10):1899-1901

[50] Green MH, Duell RM, Johnson CD, Jamieson NV. Haemobilia. The British Journal of Surgery. 2001;**88**(6): 773-786

[51] Priya H, Anshul G, Alok T, Saurabh K, Ranjit N, Romesh L, et al. Emergency cholecystectomy and hepatic arterial repair in a patient presenting with haemobilia and massive gastrointestinal haemorrhage due to a spontaneous cystic artery gallbladder fistula masquerading as a pseudoaneurysm. BMC Gastroenterology. 2013;**13**:43

[52] Hsiao CY, Kuo TC, Lai HS, Yang CY, Tien YW. Obstructive jaundice as a complication of a right hepatic artery pseudoaneurysm after laparoscopic cholecystectomy. Journal of Minimal Access Surgery. 2015;**11**(2):163-164

[53] Ouazzani A, Bataille D, Boutkhil A, Guerin E, Lefebvre JC, Vaneukem P. Spontaneous cystic artery rupture: A rare cause of haemoperitoneum. Acta Chirurgica Belgica. 2009;**109**(1):106-108

[54] Tessier DJ, Fowl RJ, Stone WM, McKusick MA, Abbas MA, Sarr MG, et al. Iatrogenic hepatic artery pseudoaneurysms: An uncommon complication after hepatic, biliary, and pancreatic procedures. Annals of Vascular Surgery. 2003;**17**(6): 663-669

[55] Choudhary A, Barakat MT, Higgins LJ, Banerjee S. Choledochoscopic identification of a hepatic/cystic artery pseudoaneurysm in a patient with hematemesis after laparoscopic cholecystectomy. Digestive Diseases and Sciences. 2017;**62**(6):1439-1442

[56] Maeda A, Kunou T, Saeki S, Aono K, Murata T, Niinomi N, et al. Pseudoaneurysm of the cystic artery with hemobilia treated by arterial embolization and elective cholecystectomy. Journal of Hepato-Biliary-Pancreatic Surgery. 2002;**9**(6):755-758

[57] Roche-Nagle G, Maceneaney, Harte P. Pseudo-aneurysm of the hepatic artery after laparoscopic cholecystectomy: A case report. Journal of Minimal Access Surgery. 2006;**2**(2):73-75

[58] Sebastian JJ, Pena E, Blas JM, Cena G. Fatal upper gastrointestinal bleeding due to hepatic artery pseudoaneurysm diagnosed by endoscopy. Digestive Diseases and Sciences. 2008;**53**(4):1152-1153

[59] Deziel DJ, Millikan KW, Economou SG, Doolas A, Ko ST, Airan MC. Complications of laparoscopic cholecystectomy: A national survey of 4,292 hospitals and an analysis of 77,604 cases. American Journal of Surgery. 1993;**165**(1):9-14

[60] Genyk YS, Keller FS, Halpern NB. Hepatic artery pseudoaneurysm and hemobilia following laser laparoscopic cholecystectomy. A case report. Surgical Endoscopy. 1994;**8**(3):201-204

[61] Saldinger PF, Wang JY, Boyd C, Lang E. Cystic artery stump pseudoaneurysm following laparoscopic cholecystectomy. Surgery. 2002;**131**(5):585-586

[62] Chen CC, Chen BB, Wang HP. Upper gastrointestinal bleeding owing to right hepatic artery pseudoaneurysm after laparoscopic cholecystectomy. Gastroenterology. 2009;**137**(5):e5-e6

[63] Boddy A, Macanovic M, Thompson J, Watkinson A. Use of an endovascular stent graft and percutaneous thrombin injection to treat an iatrogenic hepatic artery pseudoaneurysm. Annals of the Royal College of Surgeons of England. 2010;**pii**:952. DOI: 10.1308/147870810x12822015504806. ISSN: 0035-8843. https://doi.org/10.1308/147870810X12822015504806

[64] Yao CA, Arnell TD. Hepatic artery pseudoaneurysm following laparoscopic cholecystectomy. American Journal of Surgery. 2010;**199**(1):e10-e11

[65] Nakase Y, Takagi T, Fukumoto K, Kassai K, Yamagami T, Itani K, et al. Hemobilia and cystic artery stump pseudoaneurysm associated with liver abscess after a laparoscopic cholecystectomy: Report of a case. Surgery Today. 2008;**38**(6):567-571

[66] Murugesan SD, Sathyanesan J, Lakshmanan A, Ramaswami S, Perumal S, Perumal SU, et al. Massive hemobilia: A diagnostic and therapeutic challenge. World Journal of Surgery. 2014;**38**(7):1755-1762

[67] Feng W, Yue D, Zai Ming L, Zhao Yu L, Wei L, Qiyong G. Hemobilia following laparoscopic cholecystectomy: Computed tomography findings and clinical outcome of transcatheter arterial embolization. Acta Radiologica (Stockholm, Sweden: 1987). 2017;**58**(1):46-52

[68] Hylton JR, Pevec WC. Successful treatment of an iatrogenic right hepatic artery pseudoaneurysm and stenosis with a stent graft. Journal of Vascular Surgery. 2010;**51**(6):1510-1513

[69] Halbe S, Ahmed NI, Sundar K, Sathyakumar C. Pseudoaneurysm in gall bladder fossa following laparoscopic cholecystectomy. Indian Journal of Gastroenterology: Official Journal of the Indian Society of Gastroenterology. 1999;**18**(3):122

[70] Kirschberg O, Scheding A, Saers T, Krakamp B. Detection and treatment of an aneurysma spurium of the arteria hepatica dextra after laparoscopic cholecystectomy. BMC Gastroenterology. 2013;**13**:121

[71] Gandhi V, Doctor N, Marar S, Nagral A, Nagral S. Major hemobilia—Experience from a specialist unit in a developing country. Tropical Gastroenterology: Official Journal of the Digestive Diseases Foundation. 2011;**32**(3):214-218

[72] Machado NO, Al-Zadjali A, Kakaria AK, Younus S, Rahim MA, Al-Sukaiti R. Hepatic or cystic artery pseudoaneurysms following a laparoscopic cholecystectomy: Literature review of aetiopathogenesis, presentation, diagnosis and management. Sultan Qaboos University Medical Journal. 2017;**17**(2):e135-ee46

[73] Chigot V, Lallier M, Alvarez F, Dubois J. Hepatic artery pseudoaneurysm following laparoscopic cholecystectomy. Pediatric Radiology. 2003;**33**(1):24-26